HEART RISK BOOK Produced by

the Boston University's Cardiovascular Institute, the **Heart Risk Book** is an informative guide to the dangers of heart disease, with practical information on lifestyle change to help lessen your risk.

■ This special edition is presented with the compliments of John Hancock Mutual Life Insurance Company, one of the largest, most experienced and respected names in employee benefit plan management.

■ We believe one of the best ways to help hold down rising health care costs is, quite simply, by avoiding overuse of the health care delivery system. The promotion of good health is to the benefit of us all. It's a risk worth taking.

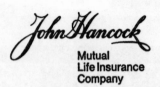

**Mutual
Life Insurance
Company**

John Hancock Place
Post Office Box 111
Boston, Massachusetts 02117

Boston University Medical Center's
HEART RISK BOOK

**A Practical Guide for
Preventing Heart Disease
by
Aram V. Chobanian, M.D.
Director, Boston University Cardiovascular
Institute
and
Lorraine Loviglio**
with Patrick O'Reilly

BANTAM BOOKS
TORONTO · NEW YORK · LONDON · SYDNEY · AUCKLAND

BOSTON UNIVERSITY MEDICAL CENTER'S
HEART RISK BOOK
A Bantam Book / June 1982

ISBN 0-553-20669-9

Published simultaneously in the United States and Canada

Bantam Books are published by Bantam Books, Inc. Its trademark,
consisting of the words "Bantam Books" and the portrayal of a rooster,
is Registered in U.S. Patent and Trademark Office and in other countries.
Marca Registrada. Bantam Books, Inc., 666 Fifth Avenue, New York,
New York 10103.

Contents

ACKNOWLEDGMENTS

Boston University Medical Center's Heart Risk Book is an expanded version of a special issue of *Bostonia*, the alumni magazine of Boston University, which appeared in 1978 under the title "What's Your Risk?" Daniel J. Finn, the University's vice president for University Relations, had suggested the special issue as a service to alumni.

It was so enthusiastically received that we decided to expand the text to book length and bring it up to date to reflect the many rapid developments in heart disease treatment and research over the past four years. Contributing to that decision was Gerald J. Gross, the University's vice president for the Arts, Publication and Media. Others from Boston University who lent support to the project were Dr. John R. Silber, president; Dr. Richard H. Egdahl, director of the Medical Center; and Dr. John I. Sandson, dean of the Medical School.

We are particularly grateful to Donald R. Giller, director of Marketing and Public Affairs for the Medical Center, who managed the project throughout, and Owen J. McNamara, director of the Medical Center's Office of Informational Services, who furnished valuable editorial support.

Finally, we are deeply indebted to Mark Kelly and to Marcia Williams, of the Educational Media Support Center of Boston University School of Medicine, for their excellent illustrations.

A.V.C.
L.W.L.

Preface

Scientific evidence accumulated over the past several years has led to the prediction that if Americans could be persuaded to lower their cardiovascular risk factors by appropriate changes in life-style and by medications, the results would be a decrease in the rate of heart attack and stroke and an increase of average life expectancy. The most recent statistics would seem to confirm this optimistic belief. Deaths from heart attacks, strokes, and other cardiovascular diseases have decreased by more than 20 percent during the past decade, and the reduction has exceeded 200,000 deaths per year. The U.S. Census Bureau has recently announced that the life expectancy for a baby girl born today is eighty-one years, and for a baby boy, seventy-two. These figures represent an increase of four years of life expectancy for females and three for males since the last figures were published. Thus, we may finally be seeing a reversal of the trend for increasing cardiovascular deaths that had been evident for the past century. Why the improvement?

A number of factors are probably involved in the drop in death rate from cardiovascular disease. Better control of high blood pressure is one obvious factor, and perhaps the most important one. Prevention of rheumatic fever and rheumatic heart disease by early treatment of streptococcal infections is another, as is new surgery for diseases of the heart valves and congenital heart disease. The introduction of coronary-care units and cardiopulmonary resuscitation for treatment of acute heart attacks has also probably had an effect. Recently it was announced by the National Heart, Lung, and Blood Institute that the average American's blood cholesterol level had dropped by 5 to 10 percent since the early 1960's, and that adults were now smoking less. These decreases may well have helped cause the sharp drop in deaths. Dr. Robert I. Levy, until recently the Institute's director, said, "What we think we are seeing now are the effects of great changes in life-styles of men and women who have been reading and listening.''

Despite these improvements, which should be the cause for great optimism, this disease is still by far the most important health problem in our country. We should not ease up, but rather intensify our efforts to combat the number-one killer. No one should feel helpless. There *are* things you can do to reduce your risk of heart attack and stroke and to protect your children. You can lose weight and limit your family's intake of calories, saturated fats, and cholesterol. You can stop smoking and see to it that your children never start. You can have your blood pressure checked; if it is high, follow your doctor's directions faithfully. You can get some exercise regularly, preferably one of the aerobic exercises such as walking, jogging, swimming, or bicycling.

The most important preventive measures you can take, and the ones with the greatest potential payoff, will be those that affect your children. If a low-fat diet, regular exercise, and health habits are made a part of daily life in your home, your children will grow up taking these things for granted, and won't have to struggle to change their habits in mid-life. And they will have a better chance of being healthy and living longer.

As a parent you can also try to influence your local school board to place more emphasis on teaching children about health and the human body. Few schools have recognized that teaching children about their own body systems is as important a part of the science curriculum as botany or chemistry. Most of our children are in danger of growing up in ignorance of how their cardiovascular system functions and how their life-style can influence their health. Yet diseases of the heart and blood vessels are the most important medical problems these children are likely to face in a few years as young adults. Heart disease is the major cause of death in males at age forty, and, some figures show, as early as age thirty. For a teenager, age thirty is not so far off.

The advances that have been made in our understanding of the causes and treatment of cardiovascular diseases during the past three decades have been truly amazing. We look forward to the future with great optimism and are certain that major steps toward the prevention and control of cardiovascular diseases will be achieved. However, there can be no progress without both major research efforts and nationwide programs to alter the life-styles of our people. The potential benefits of such efforts are immense, not only with respect to improved life expectancy but also in terms of important economic gains and a better quality of life.

Aram V. Chobanian, M.D.
Director, Boston University
Cardiovascular Institute

Procrastination versus Prevention

Why paying attention *now* to the issues raised in this book could be worth twenty extra good years of life to you

Is this you? You put antifreeze in your car *after* the temperature goes below zero. You buy snow tires *after* the first heavy snow. If so, then maybe you're also the type who thinks heart attack and stroke won't happen to you—not for a long time, anyway, and you'll have plenty of time later to do something about it.

You worry? You've never had a day of serious sickness. Even though you haven't had a checkup in ten years, you figure you're the picture of health. A little flabby, maybe, but . . . Let the other guy worry. Things happen to him, not to you.

Well, just think about it for a minute. With more than half of all deaths in the United States resulting from cardiovascular disease, there must be a lot of "other guys" around. Can you really afford to assume you'll never be one of them?

Preventing heart attack and stroke, the two major complications of atherosclerosis, takes work—a conscious, willing effort on your part. It's difficult to stick with, and you can never really know for sure whether you're a potential victim. But think about it. Isn't prevention better than treatment?

If you face the problem squarely and do something about it, you may save yourself twenty or more years of life, during which time you can accomplish a great deal for yourself, your family, and your community. Are those twenty years worth saving? If you say yes, this book is for you. It tells you:

- what you can do about preserving those twenty years;
- what the risk factors are that help bring on heart attack and stroke;
- what to do if you have a heart attack or stroke; and
- how to reduce risk factors in your children.

First, though, it will be useful to consider briefly how your cardiovascular system functions normally, what blood pressure is and how it is measured, how atherosclerosis can build up in your arteries, and what really happens when the dreaded consequences of such a build-up occur, whether in the form of angina, heart attack, stroke or sudden death.

The Cardiovascular System

The cardiovascular system consists of the heart and all the blood vessels in the body—arteries, veins, and capillaries. Arteries carry oxygen-rich blood away from the heart to the rest of the body. Veins carry the blood from which the oxygen has been removed back to the heart, which pumps it to the lungs to be replenished with oxygen. The tiny capillaries—with walls so thin that nourishment and oxygen in the blood can pass through the cells around them—are the bridges between the veins and the arteries.

Blood leaving the heart goes first into the aorta, the largest artery in the body. From there it passes into smaller and smaller arteries and arterioles (the smallest arterial branches) until it reaches its destination—for instance, the end of the big toe. At this point, the blood is traveling in a capillary, a vessel so small it cannot be seen by the naked eye. It is here that the blood nourishes the cells next to the capillary and takes away the waste products.

Having lost its oxygen and food, the blood now moves into a small vein, and from there goes to larger and larger veins; it finally flows into one large vein that receives all the blood from the lower part of the body, and from there returns to the heart.

The large artery leading from the heart is the aorta; the coronary arteries branch off from the aorta close to where it originates in the heart. The coronary arteries supply blood to the heart in the same way that the arm vessels supply blood to the hand. It is the coronary arteries which, when blocked, fail to supply the heart with enough oxygen-rich blood to sustain life.

CARDIOVASCULAR SYSTEM

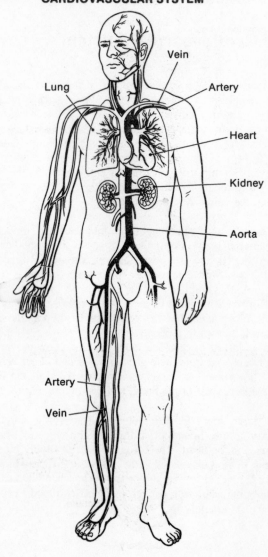

CIRCULATION THROUGH HEART

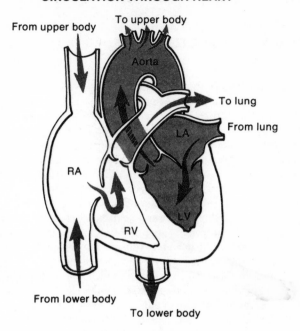

ARTERY-CAPILLARY-VEIN CIRCULATION

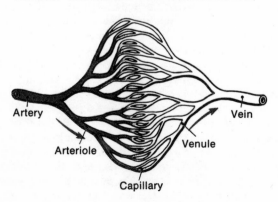

Blood Pressure

As blood flows through your body, it exerts force against the walls of the arteries. Arterial walls are elastic and muscular. They stretch and contract to take the ups and downs of blood pressure. Each time the heart beats, blood pressure in the arteries increases; each time the heart relaxes between beats, blood pressure goes down. Thus there is an upper (or systolic) and a lower (or diastolic) blood pressure, and both pressures are measured when you are examined.

Having your blood pressure measured is simple. Your nurse or doctor should measure your blood pressure routinely when you go for your annual or periodic physical. You can even do it yourself at home, with your own blood-pressure-measuring device. The device is a sphygmomanometer (sfig-moe-muh-NOM-et-er), one part of which is a rubber bag that holds air and is enclosed in a bandagelike cloth, or cuff. The doctor or nurse wraps this cuff around your arm, and uses a squeeze bulb to pump air into the cuff, which is connected to a pressure meter. He slowly releases the air and uses a stethoscope to listen to the blood flowing in your arm. When he first hears the sound of the blood surging through, he reads the meter. He reads it again when the sound ceases.

The first reading gives the systolic pressure, which indicates the greatest pressure your vessels encounter. The diastolic pressure is listed after the systolic and shows the least pressure. A systolic reading of 120 coupled with a diastolic reading of 85 would be expressed as 120/85, or 120 over 85.

For adults, the normal reading when the heart pumps—the systolic pressure—is generally between 100 and 140. The normal reading when the heart rests—the diastolic pressure—is between 70 and 90. Thus, doctors usually consider a blood-pressure reading under 140/90 normal for adults; a reading between that and 160/95 is mild high blood pressure; anything higher than that is clearly high blood pressure. Of course, these distinctions are arbitrary, since no one can say exactly at what point blood pressure becomes too high for a given individual, any more than one can give a specific weight at which a person becomes too obese.

Young, healthy people have a numerical difference ranging from 30 to 60 between their systolic and diastolic pressures. In old age, the difference can run past 100. This is because, in youth, blood vessels have a natural elasticity, which affords a degree of shock absorption to the pressure on the blood vessels. The better the shock absorption, the smoother the blood flow. The elasticity of the vessels decreases as you get older, and your vessels harden, becoming less able to withstand the pumping pressure. Thus, the force and relaxation of each spurt of blood becomes more pronounced.

In recent years, machines that measure your blood pressure automatically have become a fairly common feature in supermarkets and shopping malls. The trouble with such devices is not so much that they are inaccurate—most aren't—but that their use in a setting so different from the usual medical one tends to skew the results. In your doctor's office, you have usually been seated and quiet for some time before your blood pressure is measured. In the shopping mall or market, by contrast, you are likely to have been engaged in brisk activity right up to the time the measurement is taken, and that can throw your reading off considerably, usually causing it to be higher than usual. If you have been advised to monitor your blood pressure, don't depend on such marketplace devices to help you do the job. Instead, see your doctor, go to a clinic, or take your own reading at home.

Atherosclerosis

Atherosclerosis is silent and hidden, but is nonetheless deadly. With its complications, it represents the major cause of death in Western society. You know atherosclerosis better by the names of its two major complications: heart attack—the number-one killer in the United States—and stroke.

Atherosclerosis is the process responsible for the narrowing that may occur in arteries that supply blood to the body's vital organs. It develops when fatty materials in the blood build up in the inner wall of the arteries. The fatty deposits thicken and harden the artery, reducing its elasticity and narrowing the path through which the blood flows. If they clog a vessel so severely as to cut off blood flow entirely, the organ of the body dependent on this blood supply dies.

There is death of heart tissue (myocardial infarction), death of brain tissue (stroke, or cerebral infarction), or, occasionally, gangrene of the hands and feet.

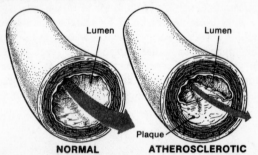

Diagrams show cross-sectional views of (A) a normal coronary artery of a person who died, and (B) a severely diseased coronary artery of a middle-aged man who died of a heart attack. Note the large opening or lumen through which blood was able to flow freely in the normal artery, and the markedly reduced lumen, which has been largely replaced by an atherosclerotic plaque, in the diseased artery.

A few years ago, doctors were predicting that if we could fight atherosclerosis effectively, we could probably eventually raise the average life expectancy by seven years. As it turns out, that prediction may have been too conservative. Recently the Census Bureau announced that, since 1950, life expectancy has already increased by four years for women and by nearly four for men. The increase was attributed primarily to a decline in the number of people dying of heart attacks and strokes. In fact, during the eight-year period from 1968 to 1976, there was approximately a 21-percent reduction in the death rate from heart attacks and an even greater decrease in mortality from strokes.

Angina, Heart Attack, and Sudden Death

The coronary arteries, those vessels carrying oxygen to the heart, are especially prone to blockage, or occlusion. Very often, people with disease of the coronary artery (generally from atherosclerosis) experience a premonition of heart attack in the form of angina pectoris, which is usually felt as a pressure sensation or pain under the breastbone or on the left side of the chest, with occasional spread of the pain to the arms or neck. Angina is your heart's way of crying out, telling you it's getting too little oxygen because of blockage or narrowing of a vessel or vessels leading to it. Unlike other types of chest pain, angina generally occurs during physical exertion or excitement, when the heart is demanding more oxygen than usual. It subsides when the exertion and excitement cease.

Prolonged angina may indicate a heart attack, or myocardial infarction. With a heart attack, so little of the required oxygen and other nutrients reach the heart that part of the heart muscle dies.

Heart attacks may produce death suddenly and without apparent warning. Half of all fatalities from heart attacks occur rather suddenly, and of these, half occur with no prior evidence of cardiac disorder. Most heart attacks are preceded by some symptoms, but the victim often fails to recognize the warning. The symptoms are often attributed to indigestion or some other relatively benign cause, either through sincere confusion or in denial of something so frightening the victim cannot admit it is happening. In perhaps one out of every ten patients, a heart attack passes completely unrecognized, with the result that the victim may later suffer a second—and possibly fatal—attack.

While part of the heart muscle is destroyed by a heart attack, there usually is more than enough normal heart muscle

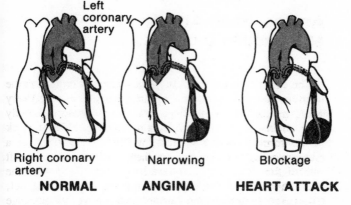

Left coronary artery

Right coronary artery

NORMAL

Narrowing

ANGINA

Blockage

HEART ATTACK

remaining after the attack to support life. What often causes heart-attack death is in reality a disturbance in the heart's electrical activity, resulting from the damage to the heart. The message that tells the heart muscle to contract in a rhythmic and synchronous way is transmitted by electrical impulses to each of the many thousand muscle fibers. When an area of the heart is damaged—as it is in a heart attack—these messages may be interrupted or distorted, causing the heart to stop beating (cardiac arrest) or the muscle to contract in an irregular, uncoordinated way (fibrillation). Swift action to correct the electrical disturbance and restore normal heartbeats—as for example through cardiopulmonary resuscitation (see pages 84–86)—can mean the difference between life and death for many heart-attack victims.

Coronary heart disease is the biggest medical threat faced by middle-aged people. Men under fifty suffer five to ten times as many heart attacks as do premenopausal women, which is why much of the research and literature concentrates on male subjects. After menopause, however, the heart-attack rate for women jumps dramatically, and by age sixty and after, the rates for both sexes become similar. No explanation has yet been found for the generally lower incidence of heart attack in premenopausal women or for the drop in the male-female ratio after age fifty.

Stroke

There are two major types of stroke: atherosclerotic brain infarction (the more common of the two) and intracranial hemorrhage, which is bleeding into the substance of the brain. Atherosclerotic brain infarction involves blockage of the blood vessels to the brain, causing death to the section of the brain deprived of oxygen. Intracranial hemorrhage occurs when disease-weakened or congenitally weak blood vessels rupture. Hypertension, or high blood pressure, is the cause of the vast majority of intracranial hemorrhages. About 95 percent of intracranial-hemorrhage victims die; most victims of atherosclerotic brain infarction may live a few years longer. With both types of stroke, at least half of those who survive their first stroke episode are left with some permanent disability.

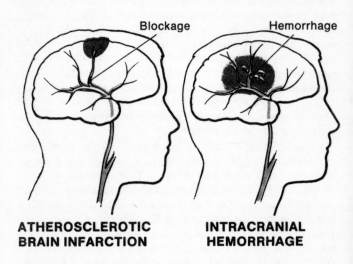

Blockage   Hemorrhage

ATHEROSCLEROTIC BRAIN INFARCTION   **INTRACRANIAL HEMORRHAGE**

Stroke's counterpart of angina—its "premonition"—is transient cerebral ischemia, which is caused by partial blockage of blood vessels carrying oxygen to the brain. Lacking sufficient oxygen, the brain will inform you by triggering certain neurologic symptoms or signs—such as slurred speech, dizziness, numbness, or weakness of the limbs—which may pass in a few minutes or a few hours. Almost always, such "little strokes" are followed eventually by a full-blown stroke, in which the blood supply to a part of the brain is completely cut off for a prolonged period, causing the death of that part of the brain deprived of oxygen and accompanying neurologic disorders that do not subside.

RISK FACTORS:
An Introduction

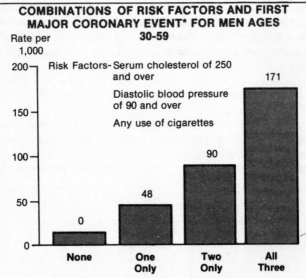

COMBINATIONS OF RISK FACTORS AND FIRST MAJOR CORONARY EVENT* FOR MEN AGES 30-59

Rate per 1,000

Risk Factors- Serum cholesterol of 250 and over

Diastolic blood pressure of 90 and over

Any use of cigarettes

Combination of major Risk Factors

None	One Only	Two Only	All Three
0	48	90	171

Hypertensives--people with significantly elevated blood pressure are four times more prone to stroke than people with normal blood pressure; diabetic hypersensitive, six times. People with normal blood pressure seldom get strokes.

Graph illustrates the increased risk of a coronary event* with the presence of one or more risk factors. For example, with no risk factors present, the rate is 20 events per 1,000 people, while with the three risk factors present the rate is 171 events per 1,000 people.

* A coronary event is defined as any clinically significant manifestation of coronary artery disease, such as heart attack or angina.

Adapted from American Heart Association, Monograph 60, 1978.

Risk factors are your habits and the facts about your physical condition that increase your chances of suffering heart attack or stroke. The three most prominent risk factors are hypertension, high cholesterol levels in the blood, and cigarette smoking. Others—considered less important because they occur less frequently, they involve less risk, or there is controversy over the role they play—include diabetes, obesity, physical activity, behavior type, salt intake (a risk factor for hypertension), and genetic and environmental factors. All will be discussed in these pages, as will the effects of drinking coffee and alcoholic beverages.

Having only one of the major risk factors at least doubles your risk of heart attack or stroke. If you have two, your risk is at least quadrupled. And having all three risk factors increases your risk to greater than eight times that of a person with none of the factors.

Hypertensives—people with significantly elevated blood pressure—are four times more prone to stroke than people with normal blood pressure; diabetic hypertensives, six times. People with normal blood pressure seldom get strokes.

RISK FACTORS: THE BIG THREE

1. High Blood Pressure

High blood pressure, or hypertension, is the most important risk factor for heart attack and stroke. It is especially significant for stroke: more than 90 percent of people who suffer strokes have high blood pressure; further, reduction of blood pressure leads to a marked decrease in the rate of strokes—even among groups of people who have already had strokes.

The only way to tell whether you have hypertension is by having your blood pressure taken. Usually, a person with hypertension has no symptoms. Your first symptoms could occur when you have a heart attack or stroke, but at that point your condition has developed into something much worse than high blood pressure, and it's much more difficult to deal with.

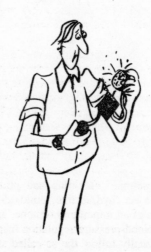

"Hypertension" is a word that misleads many people because it seems to imply, falsely, a condition brought about by being "hyper" or "tense." Hypertension is *not* nervous tension; there is no established relationship between hypertension and being strained or "uptight"; conversely, a relaxed, easygoing manner is no guarantee against high blood pressure. Neither does hypertension usually show itself through sweating, a flushed face, or dizziness. The incidence of hypertension doesn't, in most cases, correlate with particular occupations or life-styles. You don't have to be an executive or operate on a harried schedule to get it. Stress or crisis can raise blood pressure temporarily, but the pressure generally would be expected to return to its normal level once the crisis is resolved. Many experts believe that a stressful situation that exists constantly might have a deleterious effect on blood pressure, but this is not known for sure.

What we do know about hypertension is that it leads to strokes, heart attacks, heart failure, kidney failure, and other vascular complications. Hypertension can affect the circulation of any organ, since it can cause the very small arteries (arterioles) throughout the body to become narrowed.

The higher the blood pressure—systolic, diastolic, or both—the greater the risk of heart attack and stroke, as well as of heart failure, kidney failure, and impaired circulation to the extremities.

We also know that hypertension can be controlled through diet, drugs, or even surgery. Thirty years ago, control of blood pressure was possible for very few patients. Today, thanks to the extremely effective medications currently available to treat hypertension, almost every patient's blood pressure can be reduced to normal. These medications can be grouped into four classes; those that stimulate the elimination of salt by the kidneys (diuretics); those that act on the nervous system to influence its regulation of blood pressure (beta-blockers, methyldopa, reserpine, clonidine and prazosin); those that dilate blood vessels (hydralazine, minoxidil); and those that block formation of an important hormone, angiotensin, which is involved in blood-pressure regulation (captopril).

Physicians usually follow the so-called step-care approach

to treatment, in which the mildest drugs are given first and then combined, if necessary, with other, stronger medications that act differently on blood pressure. Although side effects from these medications can occur, they generally can be kept to a minimum when the drugs are used appropriately. It is extremely important for patients to continue taking their medication, even when they feel well; if they stop, their blood pressure will return to its previous high levels.

Most people with high blood pressure have only mildly elevated pressures—often only 10 to 15 points above normal. In such mild cases, medication may not be necessary. Instead, the physician may recommend that the patient lose weight, eliminate salt from his diet, engage in regular moderate exercise, and reduce stress where possible.

What doctors haven't found out yet is how, in the majority of patients, hypertension develops in the first place. Only about 10 percent of all cases of hypertension can be traced to a specific cause, such as kidney or endocrine (hormonal) disease. The remaining 90 percent of cases are called "essential hypertension," meaning hypertension that has no known cause. Discovery of the cause of the vast majority of cases does not appear to be imminent, but heightened research efforts across the country have led to many important findings in this area. And while they do not yet understand fully the underlying causes, doctors do have the ability now to lower blood pressure in almost every person with hypertension.

There is one important curable cause of hypertension that is becoming increasingly common: the use of oral contraceptive drugs. It has been discovered in recent studies that up to 5 percent of young or middle-aged women who have been on long-term treatment with oral contraceptive drugs have developed high blood pressure. Hypertension caused by these drugs can, in some cases, be very severe, but the problem generally disappears when use of the contraceptives is discontinued.

More than 35 million Americans—or better than one out of seven—have high blood pressure. If you are black, your chances of having hypertension are doubled; about 20 to 30 percent of adult blacks have the disease. Current research hopes to discover why this is true and why blacks have a

35 MILLION HYPERTENSIVES

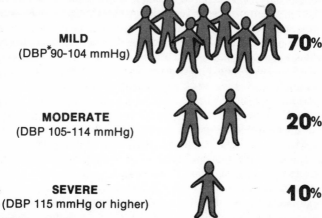

MILD
(DBP*90-104 mmHg)   **70**%

MODERATE
(DBP 105-114 mmHg)   **20**%

SEVERE
(DBP 115 mmHg or higher)   **10**%

* DBP = Diastolic blood pressure

Adapted from data of the Hypertension Detection Follow-Up Program, *J. Am. Med. Assoc.,* **242:2562-2577, 1979.**

lower incidence of heart attack, but a higher incidence of stroke, than whites.

Women have as much hypertension as men, and suffer as many strokes; however, for reasons not yet known, they suffer only a fraction of the number of heart attacks men do.

Hypertension tends to run in families, and there is evidence, based in part on research on identical twins raised apart, that the tendency is rooted more in genetics than environment. Such an inborn predisposition to develop hypertension may be a very important factor, and it may be triggered in the individual by other factors, such as overweight, high-salt diet, or oral contraceptive drugs. Other people, however, may inherit constitutional characteristics that protect them from hypertension. They may be compared to the lucky people who eat lots of fatty foods and never record high serum-cholesterol (cholesterol in the blood) levels, or who appear to indulge in high-calorie foods and yet don't gain weight.

Some studies also suggest that environment may contribute to the development of hypertension. One study noted that rural Africans who moved to cities on that continent increased their incidence of hypertension after they moved. What the studies did not show is whether the increase resulted from change in location, life-style, or diet, or was due to the upsets of urban living. Higher blood-pressure levels were also found among residents of so-called high-stress neighborhoods in Detroit, compared with residents of low-stress areas.

In 1970, several studies revealed that only about half of those who had hypertension knew of their condition, and that, of that number, only about half were receiving treatment. As a result of the increased use of screening programs and greater public awareness of the disease, more people who have hypertension are being identified than before; today, approximately two-thirds of hypertensives in the United States are aware of their illness and, of these, two-thirds have received treatment. But, unfortunately, the number of hypertensives who are adequately controlling their disease is not increasing at the same rate as the number being detected. The main problem in high-blood-pressure control is no longer detection, but maintenance of proper treatment for known hypertensives.

Salt and Blood Pressure

The role of salt in hypertension appears to be an important one, although just how important it is and exactly how it enhances the development of high blood pressure continue to be the subjects of controversy. The addition of salt to foods is a very recent development in the history of the human diet; for more than 99 percent of humankind's existence as a species, people ate either no salt at all or very little. (Even as recently as Roman times, salt was so rare and valuable it was used instead of money to pay Roman soldiers; hence our word "salary," from the Latin *salarium*, meaning "salt.") It may be that, from an evolutionary standpoint, the human body has not developed the ability to handle so much extra salt. A series of studies has furnished convincing evidence that population groups that consume extremely small amounts of salt—notably in the South Pacific, Africa, and Central and South America—have almost no hypertension. Further, blood pressure does not increase with age in these populations, as it tends to do in the rest of the world.

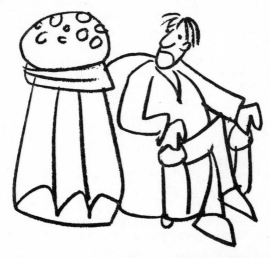

Whether the low blood pressures in those groups are simply the result of low salt intake is difficult to determine with scientific certainty; the populations involved are all unsophisticated peoples living in isolation from Western cultural influences, leaving open the possibility that other life-style differences may also be implicated. However, the low-salt groups do encompass a broad cultural spectrum, representing different races, climates, diets, customs, and methods of subsistence.

At the other end of the scale, in countries like Japan and Korea, where unusually large amounts of salt are consumed, rates of hypertension are correspondingly high. And among nomadic tribesmen in southern Iran, who also eat large amounts of salt, there is a high incidence of high blood pressure, despite the fact that the tribesmen lead strenuously active lives.

SALT INTAKE AND PREVALENCE OF HYPERTENSION

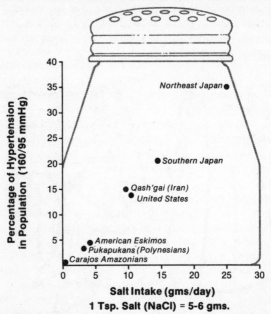

Adapted from a chapter by L. Page in *Childhood Prevention of Atherosclerosis and Hypertension*, R.M. Lauer and R.B. Shekelle, Eds., Raven Press, 1980.

Salt, or sodium chloride, contains about 40 percent sodium, and it is the sodium in salt that people with high blood pressure have to worry about. Salt is the main source of sodium in the American diet, but there are other important sources as well, including bicarbonate of soda and the food additives monosodium glutamate and sodium nitrite.

No one can say with certainty exactly how sodium affects blood pressure. One theory is that by causing excess water to be retained, sodium has the effect of expanding the body's fluid volume, thus increasing pressure within the arteries. The salt and water could also accumulate in the walls of the blood vessels themselves and increase their resistance to blood flow. A great deal of research currently focuses on the complex relationships among salt, the hormones produced by the kidneys, the function of the kidneys themselves, and the workings of the adrenal glands. These factors seem to be closely interrelated, and it is not enough to speak of the role of salt alone.

Human beings need sodium in their diet—at least 200 milligrams per day, or the equivalent of less than one-tenth of a teaspoon of salt. We Americans take in a great deal more—by some estimates, about twenty times that amount, or the equivalent of an average of two teaspoons of salt a day. Most of us realize that many of our favorite junk foods and snacks are heavily salted, but few are probably aware of how much salt or other sources of sodium are found in virtually every processed food on supermarket shelves.

It is not necessarily the foods we ordinarily think of as salty that have the highest sodium content. A one-ounce serving of a popular brand of corn flakes, for example, contains nearly twice as much sodium as an ounce of cocktail peanuts. Two slices of a quality-brand white bread contains more sodium than a one-ounce bag of potato chips. Amazingly, pudding has more sodium than bacon: a one-half cup serving of a popular brand of chocolate-flavored instant pudding contains over 100 milligrams more sodium than three slices of bacon. A patient on a mild low-sodium diet is usually restricted to about 2,000 milligrams of sodium a day. Yet a single large dill pickle contains more than 1,000 milligrams of sodium. And if you decide to forget about the supermarket and go to your favorite fast-food restaurant, you might be worse off: a popular chain's special double hamburger comes loaded with 1,510 milligrams of sodium—roughly three-quarters of the daily allotment for a patient on a low-salt diet.

Until recently, even baby foods were heavily salted to appeal to what was presumed to be the mother's taste. Now baby-food manufacturers seem to have responded to increased consumer awareness by cutting down or eliminating salt from their products.

Many people appear to suffer no ill effects from a diet high in salt; they are believed by most authorities on hypertension to be resistant to the disease. Other people seem to inherit a susceptibility to hypertension; in them, a high-salt diet appears

COMPARISON OF SODIUM CONTENT IN COMMONLY USED FOODS

	LOW			HIGH	
	Portion	Sodium (mg)		Portion	Sodium (mg)
DAIRY					
Natural Swiss Cheese	1 oz.	74	Pasteurized Process Swiss	1 oz.	388
Low-fat Milk	1 cup	122	Canned Evaporated Skim Milk	1 cup	294
Lo-Cal Pudding	½ cup	115	Instant Whole Milk Pudding	½ cup	470
FISH, MEAT & POULTRY					
Canned Salmon, no salt added	3 oz.	41	Canned Salmon, salt added	3 oz.	443
Raw Shrimp	3 oz.	137	Canned Shrimp	3 oz.	1,955
Cooked Lean Beef	3 oz.	55	Cooked Corned Beef	3 oz.	802
Fresh, Cooked Lean Ham	3 oz.	59	Cured Ham	3 oz.	1,114
BEANS AND NUTS					
Dry Cooked Kidney Beans	1 cup	4	Canned Kidney Beans	1 cup	844
Unsalted Peanuts	1 cup	8	Dry Roasted, Salted Peanuts	1 cup	986
VEGETABLES					
Raw Carrots	1 carrot	34	Carrots, Frozen in Butter Sauce	3.3 oz.	350
Corn, Frozen	1 cup	7	Canned Whole Kernel Corn	1 cup	384
Mushrooms, Raw	1 cup	7	Canned Mushrooms	2 oz.	242
Cooked Green Peas	1 cup	2	Canned Peas	1 cup	493
Raw Tomatoes	1 tomato	14	Canned Whole Tomatoes	1 cup	390
CONDIMENTS					
Garlic Powder	1 tsp.	1	Garlic Salt	1 tsp.	1,850
Low Sodium Meat Tenderizer	1 tsp.	1	Regular Meat Tenderizer	1 tsp.	1,750
Oil & Vinegar	1 tbsp.	1	Bottled Italian Salad Dressing	1 tbsp.	116

from: *The Sodium Content of Your Food, U.S. Dept. of Agriculture. Home & Garden Bulletin #233, 1980.*

to trigger the disease. If there is high blood pressure in your family, you have some reason to suspect that you might be one of the susceptible people. Unfortunately, there is no good way to know for sure. The prudent course, therefore, seems to be to play it safe by limiting your salt intake to small amounts throughout your life. In any case, the evidence strongly suggests that salt should certainly be used sparingly by people who are already hypertensive.

Besides its potential for aggravating the disease, a high salt intake can block the blood-pressure-lowering effect of medications, especially diuretics, or make it necessary for the patient to take larger doses of drugs, thereby increasing his or her chances of experiencing side effects. Salt should also be used in very small quantities by anyone with heart disease, and by those who are likely to be susceptible to hypertension—black people, obese people, and especially people with kidney disease or a family history of hypertension.

Genetic and Environmental Factors

Race and geography affect blood-pressure levels, scientists have observed, though they haven't been able to discover why. Are the differences genetic, dietary, or environmental? Theories differ. There is evidence that hypertension tends to run in families. But in the case of geography, at least, it seems likely that it is the differing life-styles of certain countries and regions, rather than innate characteristics, that account for observed differences.

About 25 to 30 percent of the black adults in the United States have hypertension, compared with about 15 percent of white adults. Some inconclusive differences in hypertension rates have been found from one section of the country to another, but the incidence of hypertension among blacks is higher than among whites in all regions.

Some studies have attempted to link the higher incidence of hypertension in blacks to life-style and environmental factors. Since large numbers of blacks have low incomes and live in unfavorable circumstances—especially in the inner city—stress has been thought by some to play a possible role in black people's high rate of hypertension. So far, no study has succeeded in singling out any consistent habits or environmental characteristics to which elevated blood pressure could be attributed. However, two recently published studies—one in California and the other in South Carolina—provide additional evidence that environmental factors, and especially social class, may play a significant role in the development of blood pressure. The California study showed that both blacks and whites from low-income, low-status residential areas had the highest blood pressure readings and that low social status was a more important risk factor for hypertension than being black. In South Carolina, researchers discovered that dark skin pigmentation was not as important a factor for hypertension as was low social status.

The idea that job-related stress might increase the risk of hypertension received a significant boost when a study conducted at Boston University Medical Center showed that air-traffic controllers had four times the rate of hypertension as the population at large (see discussion, page 72).

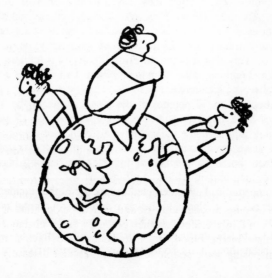

2. Cholesterol

A high level of lipids (fats) in the blood and blood vessels is second only to hypertension as a major risk factor for atherosclerosis and coronary heart disease.

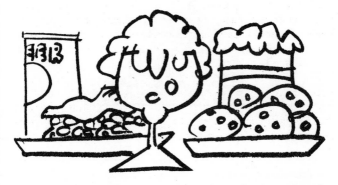

As we saw earlier in the discussion of atherosclerosis, lipids flowing through the body in the bloodstream may be deposited in the walls of the blood vessels and cause narrowing, scarring, and stiffening. Narrowed vessels may prevent blood from getting through adequately.

Of the several types of fatty materials in the blood, cholesterol is the most widely studied and is best known to the public. A normal part of blood and all body tissue, cholesterol is essential for the synthesis of certain important hormones. You get some of your cholesterol from the foods you eat, but your liver and other tissues produce it, too—even if you have *no* cholesterol in your diet. If there is too much of this fatlike substance in your bloodstream, it can contribute to the clogging of your arteries and increase your risk of heart attack. (Triglycerides, another group of fatty substances that circulate in the blood, are also believed to have a role in predisposing some people to develop vascular disease.)

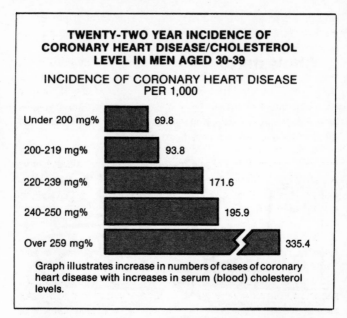

TWENTY-TWO YEAR INCIDENCE OF CORONARY HEART DISEASE/CHOLESTEROL LEVEL IN MEN AGED 30-39

INCIDENCE OF CORONARY HEART DISEASE PER 1,000

Under 200 mg% 69.8

200-219 mg% 93.8

220-239 mg% 171.6

240-250 mg% 195.9

Over 259 mg% 335.4

Graph illustrates increase in numbers of cases of coronary heart disease with increases in serum (blood) cholesterol levels.

Adapted from T.R. Dawber, *Current Concepts*, Upjohn, 1975.

Recently, some important new light has been shed on the cholesterol picture with the discovery of what has been popularly described as "good cholesterol" and "bad cholesterol." To be dissolved in the blood, cholesterol has to be bound to a protein; the resulting substance is a lipoprotein, and several types normally exist in the blood. What recent studies have discovered is that these lipoproteins include two major types that have opposite effects on the arteries: high-density lipoprotein (HDL), which may protect against atherosclerosis, and low-density lipoprotein (LDL), which may promote development of the disease. Persons whose HDL cholesterol is relatively high have less risk of developing coronary heart disease, while people with a high LDL level have a greater risk. (The role of a third component, very low-density lipoprotein, or VLDL, is still unclear, but it appears to precede and give rise to LDL and may itself be harmful if present in excess. Triglycerides are transported in the bloodstream predominantly by VLDLs.)

The reason for HDL's protective effect is uncertain, but it may be that HDL picks up cholesterol from arteries and other body cells and transports it to the liver, where it can be metabolized or excreted. By carrying cholesterol away from artery-wall cells, HDL may discourage the development of atherosclerotic plaques.

Studies of families in which one generation after another has lived to age 80 or 90 without cardiovascular disease have revealed that family members had either very high HDL levels or very low levels of LDL. Women have a higher average level of HDL than men, possibly explaining, to some extent, women's relative immunity to cardiovascular disease. Researchers have also found that marathon runners, and even joggers, have higher HDL levels than inactive people (see "Exercise," page 57).

Can you do anything, short of becoming a long-distance runner, to raise the level of HDL in your blood and lower the supply of LDL? Scientists are now trying to find an answer to that question, and research is under way to try to develop drugs that would create a more favorable balance between the two components. In the meantime, any measure of your blood cholesterol, to be meaningful, should include an assessment of total cholesterol and HDL to determine your risk of coronary heart disease.

The Importance of Diet

One thing you can do that may help to keep fatty materials from lodging in your blood vessels is to reduce the amount of fat in your diet. It's true that high blood cholesterol is partly a problem of body chemistry: some people can eat a high-fat, high-cholesterol diet and still have normal blood-cholesterol levels, while the body chemistry of other people keeps their cholesterol levels high despite even the most stringent diet. Nevertheless, the vast majority of Americans who develop coronary heart disease have high levels of fats in their blood caused in large part by what they eat. Thus, a low-fat, low-cholesterol diet is recommended by most physicians. The goals of such a diet should be to (1) limit the amount of fat and saturated fat, and (2) restrict the amount of cholesterol in the diet, and (3) reduce the overall intake of calories.

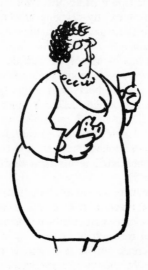

Until quite recently, scientists advised substituting polyunsaturated fats for saturated fats wherever possible, because polyunsaturated fats tend to lower blood cholesterol. Currently, however, many of these experts are less convinced that a marked increase in the use of polyunsaturates is desirable, and instead are advising people only to reduce their intake of saturated fats, pending further research.

Polyunsaturated fats are derived from vegetable products, are usually liquid at room temperature, and include such things as corn, cottonseed, soybean, and safflower oils. "Polyunsaturated" refers to the chemical structure of the fatty acid: its molecules consist of groups of carbon atoms that have fewer hydrogen atoms associated with them, and are thus said to be less hydrogenated.

Saturated fats tend to raise blood cholesterol. They are

usually fats of animal origin, and are frequently solid, rather than liquid, like the fats in butter and meat.

There are two liquid vegetable oils that are, nonetheless, highly saturated and to be avoided—palm oil and coconut oil. Both are cheap, have a long shelf life, and are increasingly used in nondairy cream substitutes, frozen desserts, and other processed foods. Cocoa butter, the fat in chocolate, is (unfortunately for many lovers of chocolate) another saturated vegetable fat that needs to be restricted. Further, some margarines soften at room temperature, even though they are hydrogenated. So it is important to read labels to identify the exact nature of the fats.

Generally speaking, a diet designed to reduce blood levels of cholesterol and to thereby help prevent atherosclerosis should limit meat consumption, eliminate such fatty meats as bacon, luncheon meats, spare ribs, and the like, and emphasize lean meat, fish, and poultry. It should also avoid or reduce the use of egg yolks, whole milk, cream and other high-fat dairy products, butter and lard, most cheeses, chocolate, and such saturated vegetable fats as coconut oil, palm oil, and cocoa butter and the products made from them, such as most simulated dairy products and certain shortenings.

Instead, the low-cholesterol diet should substitute for the prohibited foods such things as egg whites, skim milk, water ices and sherbets made with skim milk, margarine, vegetable shortenings and oils, and low-fat cottage cheese. Fish and poultry should be substituted as much as possible for red meat, because they have less saturated fats.

Foods that are by nature predominantly fat should be eaten in moderate quantities; they include margarine, shortening, oils, nuts, peanut butter, olives, and avocados. You should use sparingly such high-fat foods as bottled salad dressings, potato chips and similar snack foods, fried foods, "fancy breads," and rich desserts.

Use fruits, vegetables, whole-grain cereals, and legumes (peas and beans) to replace the high-fat, high-cholesterol foods removed from your diet.

To Americans accustomed to a diet loaded with fat and cholesterol, such a prescription may seem unnecessarily severe.

But consider that a diet high in saturated fats and cholesterol can lead through high cholesterol levels in the blood to the development of atherosclerotic plaques, and from there to a high incidence of heart attack and stroke. The intake of cholesterol in the United States, which has a very high rate of death from coronary heart disease, generally ranges between a high 600 to 1,000 milligrams per day. In Japan, where the death rate from coronary heart disease traditionally has been low, dietary cholesterol and fat have been correspondingly low.

Since high levels of cholesterol and other fats in the blood can begin to develop early in life, it is important to begin taking preventive measures in early childhood. You should follow a preventive-diet regimen not only for your own sake but especially for the sake of your children. Obviously, if you

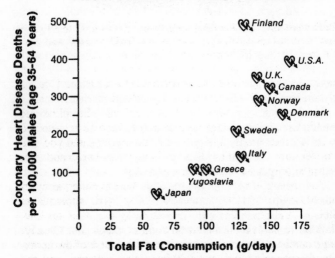

FAT CONSUMPTION AND MORTALITY FROM CORONARY HEART DISEASE

Data were obtained for men ranging in age from 35 to 64 years and were adapted from an article by O. Turpeinen, *Circulation* 59:1-7, 1979.

CHOLESTEROL INTAKE AND MORTALITY FROM CORONARY HEART DISEASE

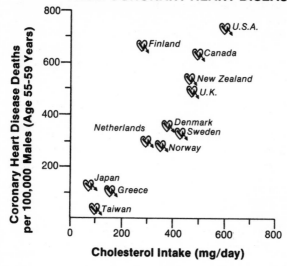

Data were obtained for men ranging in age from 55 to 59 years and were adapted from an article by W.E. Connor and S.L. Connor, *Prev. Med.* 1:49-83, 1972.

have a diagnosed problem of high blood cholesterol or triglycerides yourself, you need to follow a strict dietary plan.

The low-fat, low-cholesterol diet will take discipline and intelligence, but it becomes easier as you become accustomed to it. In time, whole milk will taste too creamy, and you will wonder how you could ever have thought that bacon and eggs were the only foods fit to begin your day.

You have probably already noticed the increasing array of substitutes for high-cholesterol foods on your supermarket shelves, and noted as well the increasing emphasis on low-cholesterol content in television food commercials. Clearly, large numbers of Americans are becoming aware of the necessity for changing old, unhealthful eating patterns, and the food processors are responding. Recently, government officials announced that the average American's cholesterol level

CHOLESTEROL AND FAT CONTENT OF FOODS

	serving size	total fat (grams)	saturated fatty acids (grams)	monounsaturated fatty acids (grams)	polyunsaturated fatty acids (grams)	cholesterol (milligrams)	food energy (calories)
Fluid whole milk	1 cup	9.0	5.0	3.0	trace	34	165
Low fat milk (1%)	1 cup	2.5	1.6	.8	trace	14	103
American cheese	1 oz.	9.0	5.0	3.0	trace	25	105
Cheddar cheese	1 oz.	9.0	5.0	3.0	trace	28	115
Cottage cheese—creamed (4% fat)	1 cup	10.0	6.0	3.0	trace	48	260
Cottage cheese—uncreamed	1 cup	1.0	trace	trace	trace	13	170
Swiss cheese	1 oz.	8.0	4.0	3.0	trace	28	105
Yogurt—plain, made from partially skimmed milk	8 oz.	4.0	2.0	1.0	trace	17	125
Ice cream—regular (approx. 10% fat)	1 cup	14.0	8.0	5.0	trace	53	255
Lean beef, lamb, pork, ham	3 oz.	8.4	3.9	3.5	trace	77	189
Lean veal	3 oz.	4.8	2.4	2.3	trace	84	177
Poultry	3 oz.	5.1	1.5	2.6	1.0	74	150
Fish	3 oz.	4.5	.9	no data	.3	63	126
Crab	½ cup	2.0	.5	.7	.8	62	85

	size serving	total fat (grams)	saturated fatty acids (grams)	monounsaturated fatty acids (grams)	polyunsaturated fatty acids (grams)	cholesterol (milligrams)	food energy (calories)
Lobster	½ cup	1.0	no data	no data	no data	62	68
Shrimp	½ cup (11 large)	1.0	.2	.3	.5	96	100
Tuna—packed in oil, drained solids	3 oz.	8.2	3.0	no data	2.0	65	197
Liver (beef)	3 oz.	3.4	no data	no data	no data	327	136
Eggs, chicken, whole	1 large	6.0	2.0	3.0	trace	250	80
Peanut butter	2 tbsp.	16.0	3.2	8.0	4.5	0	190
Butter	1 tbsp.	12.0	6.0	4.0	trace	35	100
Stick margarine	1 tbsp.	11.2	2.0	3.6	5.3	0	100
Polyunsaturated corn oil	1 tbsp.	14.0	2.0	4.0	8.0	0	125
Sunflower oil	1 tbsp.	14.0	1.6	3.9	8.5	0	125
Olive oil	1 tbsp.	14.0	2.8	7.0	3.9	0	125
Coconut oil	1 tbsp.	14.0	13.0	2.0	trace	0	125
Peanut oil	1 tbsp.	14.0	20.0	10.0	2.0	0	125

from: *American Heart Association Cookbook*, 1973, 1975.

had dropped by 5 to 10 percent since the early 1960's and said that this decrease may have contributed to a sharp drop in deaths from heart and blood-vessel diseases.

Some supermarket chains, responding to their customers' heightened health-consciousness, have begun using color codes to identify foods as being either high or low in cholesterol, sodium, or saturated fats. A few company cafeterias are furnishing the same kind of information for corporate employees. If such a service is not available to you at your supermarket or company cafeteria, you might try asking that it be introduced. One warning: Because similar food products often contain different ingredients, you should learn to read labels properly. Labels on processed foods will tell you what kinds of fat went into them and what methods of preparation were used. If you have been diagnosed as suffering from hypercholesterolemia (high blood cholesterol), you may wish to consult, in addition to your physician, a nutritionist, who will tell you what the labels don't tell you. For example, some labels list only "vegetable oil," without indicating whether the vegetable oil is saturated or polyunsaturated, so you don't know whether you're getting safflower oil (polyunsaturated) or coconut oil (saturated).

A nutritionist can also steer you in the direction of permissible replacements for "forbidden foods" or for those recommended foods that you just don't like—maybe a different brand of the product in question or a homemade version of a supermarket item. You will have to give up the rich desserts you may have been fond of, but there are recipes for good-tasting desserts you can make at home, substituting for forbidden ingredients. You can obtain these from a nutritionist or from a number of excellent cookbooks that are available, including one prepared by the American Heart Association. (See Bibliography, page 101.) These sweets often taste very much like the original dessert and can be enjoyed by everyone in the family, including the kids.

Many people have begun to enjoy a low-saturated-fat or low-cholesterol diet and have found it may be helpful in weight control by cutting down on high-calorie foods. But some of us fall prey to temptations and rationalizations: we complain that lean meat costs more than fatty meat; that the store doesn't carry a certain item; that the kids won't drink skimmed milk; that such-and-such a newspaper article conflicts with a recommendation on our diet. If you're about to stray, try to remember that, when you weigh it against the possible benefits to your health, sticking to your special diet isn't such a heavy burden, after all.

Some recent findings, suggesting that persons with very low levels of blood cholesterol may have a slightly higher risk of developing cancer, have caused some people to question the wisdom of aggressively lowering cholesterol levels. However, even if there is an increased risk, it would be very small in comparison with the potent effect of high blood cholesterol on the development of cardiovascular disease. Besides, few Americans have cholesterol levels so low that they need have any concern about increasing their risk for cancer.

Dietary Guidelines for Americans

In 1980 the U.S. Department of Agriculture and the U.S. Department of Health, Education and Welfare issued a set of dietary guidelines for Americans. The following is adapted from those official government guidelines.

1. Eat a variety of foods daily, including selections of:
   - fruits
   - vegetables
   - whole-grain and enriched breads, cereals, and grain products
   - milk, cheese, and yogurt
   - legumes (dry peas and beans)

2. Maintain ideal weight.
   If you need to lose weight, do so gradually.
   Avoid crash diets that are severely restricted in the variety of foods they allow.

3. Avoid too much fat, saturated fat, and cholesterol.
   - Choose lean meat, fish, poultry, dry beans and peas as your protein sources.
   - Moderate your use of eggs and organ meats (such as liver).
   - Limit your intake of butter, cream, hydrogenated margarines, shortenings and coconut oil, and foods made from such products.
   - Trim excess fat off meats.
   - Broil, bake, or boil rather than fry.
   - Read labels carefully to determine both amount and types of fat contained in foods.

4. Eat food with adequate starch and fiber.
   - Substitute starches for fats and sugars.
   - Select foods which are good sources of fiber and starch, such as whole-grain breads and cereals, fruits and vegetables, beans, peas, and nuts.

5. Avoid eating too much sugar, and foods high in sugar content.

6. Avoid eating too much salt (sodium) and foods high in salt.

7. If you drink alcohol, do so in moderation.

U.S. Dietary Goals

A few years ago the Select Committee on Nutrition and Human Needs of the U.S. Senate issued a report outlining dietary goals for the United States. The diagrams below illustrate the proportions of fat, protein and carbohydrate in the current average American diet, on the left, and the proportions recommended by the Senate committee, on the right.

U.S. Dietary Goals

1. Increase carbohydrate consumption to account for 55 to 60 percent of the energy (caloric) intake.
2. Reduce over all fat consumption from approximately 40 to 30 percent of energy intake.

3. Reduce saturated fat consumption to account for about 10 percent of total energy intake; and balance that with poly-unsaturated and mono-unsaturated fats, which should account for about 10 percent of energy intake each.
4. Reduce cholesterol consumption to about 300 mg. a day.
5. Reduce sugar consumption by about 40 percent to account for about 15 percent of total energy intake.
6. Reduce salt consumption by about 50 to 85 percent to approximately 3 grams a day.

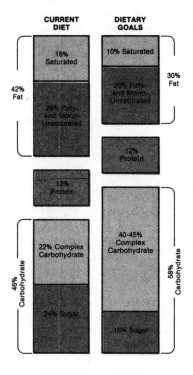

(Adapted from "Dietary Goals for the United States" second edition, prepared by the staff of the Select Committee on Nutrition and Human Needs, United States Senate, U.S. Government Printing Office, Washington, D.C., 1977.)

3. Smoking

Cigarette smoking, according to the 1979 U.S. Surgeon General's Report on Smoking and Health, is the largest preventable cause of death in America. Besides increasing the risk for lung cancer by more than twentyfold and being the principal cause of emphysema, smoking is also a villain in heart disease and stroke, for which it is one of the three biggest risk factors.

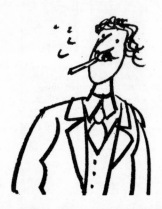

It is coronary heart disease, not lung cancer, that is the principal cause of the increased mortality rate among cigarette smokers. Of the 700,000 annual deaths from heart disease, a significant proportion are attributable to cigarette smoking. Sudden death from heart attack occurs two to three times as often among men who smoke as among those who do not.

If you smoke more than a pack a day, you increase your risk of heart disease threefold. The heightened risk among smokers for heart attack and for death following heart attack increases the longer they have smoked, the more cigarettes they smoke per day, and the more they inhale. (The risk for

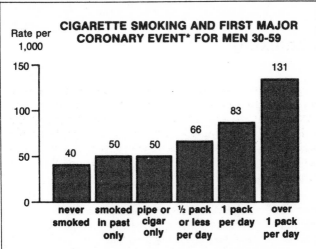

CIGARETTE SMOKING AND FIRST MAJOR CORONARY EVENT* FOR MEN 30-59

Rate per 1,000

never smoked	smoked in past only	pipe or cigar only	½ pack or less per day	1 pack per day	over 1 pack per day
40	50	50	66	83	131

Graph illustrates the varying rates of coronary events* depending upon smoking habits. For example, those men who never smoked had a rate of 40 coronary events per 1,000 individuals, while those smoking over a pack a day had a rate of 131 events per 1,000 individuals.

* A coronary event is defined as any clinically significant manifestation or coronary artery disease, such as heart attack or angina.

Adapted from American Heart Association, Monograph 60, 1978.

pipe and cigar smokers may be less, presumably because they don't inhale as much smoke.) If you survive a heart attack and keep on smoking, you increase your chances of having a second attack. The effect of smoking, when combined with other risk factors—such as hypertension or high cholesterol—is not additive, but compounded.

Autopsy studies have established that atherosclerosis—the process by which arteries become narrow through the buildup of fatty material on their inner walls—is more severe and extensive in smokers than in nonsmokers. Again, the more you smoke, the more severe your atherosclerosis is likely to be. Smoking is also a major risk factor for arteriosclerotic peripheral vascular disease (atherosclerosis in the limbs; see

p. 79). So far, no clear relationship has been established between smoking and stroke, but an association with a form of stroke—subarachnoid hemorrhage—has been reported in women.

Smoking can increase the pulse rate, constrict the blood vessels, and cause premature heartbeats, an irregular rhythm of the heart. A lighted cigarette gives off several hundred compounds, some of them in gaseous form, others in the form of particles, or tar. The tar includes at least a dozen known carcinogens (cancer-producing agents), as well as nicotine, a toxic chemical; the gases include carbon monoxide, ammonia, and hydrogen cyanide, among others. Scientists still don't know whether the culprit in cigarette smoke is nicotine, carbon monoxide, some other ingredient, or a combination of ingredients. Similarly, whether or not filters are effective in minimizing the toxic effects of smoking is not yet clear. The most recent data suggest that people who smoke filtered cigarettes have about the same incidence of coronary disease as smokers who indulge in nonfiltered cigarettes.

According to the Surgeon General's report, smokers of cigarettes low in tar and nicotine may have a lower risk for coronary heart disease than those smoking high-tar, high-nicotine cigarettes, but that risk may still be considerably greater than that of nonsmokers. And for some, even the small amount of protection offered by low-tar-and-nicotine products may prove to be illusory. The heavy smoker, in an effort to keep his blood concentration of nicotine at the accustomed level, may end up smoking more of these "low-tar" cigarettes and puffing each one more often.

"Secondhand smoking"—the effects of cigarette smoke on the nonsmoker—has become the object of increased attention in recent years, as nonsmokers have begun to assert their right to breathe air unpolluted by their neighbors' cigarettes and cigars. Such involuntary smoking has been shown to cause irritation of the eyes and nose in a substantial part of the normal population. More alarming, however, is the finding that it can cause anginal attacks in people with coronary artery disease. In a study in which men with angina pectoris were given exercise after being exposed to a smoke-filled

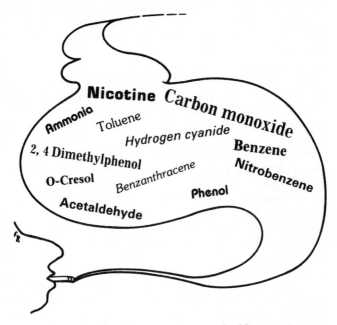

room, they were found to experience pain 38 percent sooner than after being exposed to uncontaminated air. Persons with chronic lung disease are also particularly vulnerable to the effects of involuntary smoking.

Studies of the children of parents who smoke show they are more likely to have bronchitis and pneumonia during the first year of life. Since the more the parents smoke, the higher the incidence of illness, it seems reasonable to suspect that cigarette smoke in the environment of the home is the cause of these infant infections.

Until fairly recently, most studies on the effects of smoking on health involved only men, because women didn't begin to smoke heavily and in large numbers until recent years. Perhaps because all the frightening statistics referred only to men, many women may have been lulled into a false sense that they were somehow immune to the devastating effects of smoking. Now, with the increased number of women smokers, and with the increasingly early ages at which girls begin to smoke, all that is changing. Studies published in the last few years have clearly demonstrated that for women, as for men, cigarette smoking presents serious risk to health and life.

One such study, conducted by the American Cancer Society, showed that women between the ages of forty-five and fifty-five who smoke are twice as likely as nonsmokers to die of a stroke or heart disease. Women smokers were also found to have a greater risk of dying at a young age from lung cancer, emphysema and bronchitis, cirrhosis of the liver, aortic aneurysm (a "blowout" in the body's main artery), and cancer of the mouth, pharynx, larynx, and esophagus. The risk of premature death was greatest among women who smoked the most cigarettes and who inhaled.

If you are a woman who smokes, you are approximately doubling your risk for heart disease. But if you are a young woman who both smokes and uses oral contraceptives, *you are multiplying your risk by ten*. This risk increases significantly with age, so that a woman between the ages of thirty-eight and forty-five who both smokes and takes the pill has a dangerously high risk of heart attack. The same synergistic effect—that is, where two or more risk factors combine to create a total risk greater than the sum of their individual risks—has been suggested for smoking and oral contraceptives in subarachnoid hemorrhage, a form of stroke.

Smoking carries a double threat for women—not only to their own health and life, but also to their ability to bear healthy children. Pregnant women who smoke have more miscarriages and premature births, and have more of their babies die in the first few days after delivery than do mothers who do not smoke. They also have smaller babies—weighing on the average a half-pound less than the babies of nonsmokers—and their babies suffer more health problems.

How does smoking affect the development of the fetus? Although this question has not yet been fully answered, it is known that nicotine passes into the circulation of the developing fetus from the smoking mother's blood. In addition, carbon monoxide levels have been shown to rise in the blood of the fetus; since carbon monoxide combines with the hemoglobin of red blood cells, its presence reduces the capacity of the blood to carry necessary oxygen to developing tissues.

While adults, made increasingly aware of the health hazards of smoking, have been smoking less in recent years, the same cannot be said of their teenage children. Smoking among teenage boys has remained at about the same level, and among teenage girls it is actually increasing. According to the 1979 Surgeon General's report, in the brief period between 1968 and 1974 the percentage of regular smokers among children between the ages of twelve and fourteen increased from 6 to 12 percent. The tragic implications of these statistics can be understood in light of the fact that death rates from all causes are significantly higher among people who start smoking earlier in life.

It is not ignorance that causes teenagers to take up smoking, since by the time they reach junior high school nearly all children know that smoking is dangerous. Apparently some combination of peer pressure, parental example, and the lure of advertising outweighs the threat to future health among many young people. The prevention of smoking by children is surely one of the most vital steps for their future health and well-being that we can take as parents. In addition, it is one of the most significant public-health objectives we can adopt as members of our communities.

While scientists still don't have all answers about how cigarette smoking contributes to illness and shortens life, one thing they do know for sure is that it is well worth your while to quit. When you quit smoking, almost immediately you reduce your risk of a heart attack by 50 percent. Men who quit smoking average one-third to one-half fewer heart attacks than those who don't. Furthermore, the mortality rate for male ex-smokers due to all causes drops by one-fourth. After ten years off cigarettes, your risk of dying from coronary heart disease approaches that of a nonsmoker. Obviously, the earlier you quit and the shorter the time that you have been smoking, the better your chances. But quitting smoking at any age improves health and life expectancy; it is never too late to quit.

Giving up cigarettes also helps to increase your breathing capacity and helps to make you more resistant to pneumonias and chronic bronchitis. A restricted breathing capacity also has an indirect effect on heart function by limiting the amount of exercise you get.

A smoking habit is a physical and psychological addiction that's difficult to break. Smokers often use the excuse that they shouldn't stop smoking because they'll gain weight, and they "reason" that weight is also a risk factor in heart disease. The fact of the matter is that people who quit smoking gain only a small amount of weight—usually about five to ten pounds—during the course of a year, and then their weight gain levels off. They don't continue to balloon out as the years go by. This may cause a problem with your wardrobe, but probably nothing more serious; doctors say that the risk involved in a weight gain of five to ten pounds is negligible compared to the tremendous benefits of quitting. And if you watch your diet carefully after quitting smoking, you can avoid any permanent weight gain altogether.

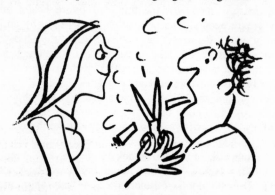

Tips to Help You Quit Smoking

1. Decide positively that you want to quit smoking. Avoid dwelling on how difficult it might be.

2. Set a target date for quitting—a special day, like your birthday, anniversary, or a holiday—but don't make it so far off that you lose momentum.
3. Begin to condition yourself physically. Start a modest exercise regimen, drink more fluids, get plenty of rest.
4. Try to gain the support of at least one other person, preferably an ex-smoker, or ask a friend or your spouse to quit with you.
5. Note the occasions when you are most apt to smoke and try to avoid these situations. For example, get up from the table directly after a meal; cut down on coffee drinking or alcohol consumption.
6. Before you quit, change your brand of cigarettes often, and buy them only by the pack. Don't store up cigarettes.
7. Smoke only enough to satisfy your craving—half a cigarette at most.
8. Each day, postpone lighting your cigarette by one hour.
9. Decide beforehand how many cigarettes you will smoke during the day. Keep a written record in the back of the pack of where, when, and how many cigarettes you smoke.
10. Give yourself a reward when you reach certain goals, and a "punishment" (e.g., a donation to charity) if you backslide.
11. Never smoke after you get a craving until *three* minutes have passed. During those three minutes change what you are doing or what you are thinking about. Or telephone a friend, especially an ex-smoker.
12. Don't carry cigarettes with you. Make them difficult to get to. Don't carry a lighter or matches.
13. Make yourself a "smoking corner" that is far away from anything pleasurable. Never smoke while watching television.
14. Think of the negative effects of smoking on your body: hot and scratchy air is going in and out of

your black and unhealthy lungs; you are exhaling an unpleasant odor, and people are turning away from you; your skin is becoming wrinkled and aged as the nicotine and carbon monoxide circulate in your body; your arteries are becoming clogged with deposits of fatty scar tissue.

15. Become involved in new activities, particularly ones requiring the use of your hands.

16. Spend as much free time as possible in places where smoking is prohibited, such as libraries, museums, stores, churches, theaters, and swimming pools. Take a shower—you can't smoke there.

17. Develop smoking substitutes; try relaxation techniques or exercise. Keep your hands busy by knitting or doing puzzles.

18. Keep oral substitutes handy, like carrots, celery, apples, raisins, sugarless gum, etc. Avoid foods that are high in calories.

19. Enjoy some new oral sensations: brush your teeth three times daily, drink large quantities of water or juice, eat new foods like raw vegetables, fruits.

20. If you're having a sudden craving for a cigarette, take ten deep breaths, holding the last while you light a match. Exhale slowly and blow out the match, crushing it out in an ashtray like a cigarette.

21. Don't be discouraged if, after an initial dramatic decrease in the amount of your smoking, you notice a temporary leveling off. Remember, quitting isn't easy, but you *can* do it.

22. Never allow yourself to think "one won't hurt." It will.

From: *Calling It Quits*, U.S. Department of Health, Education and Welfare, Publication No. (NIH) 79-1824.

Tip Sheet, American Cancer Society, Massachusetts Division, Inc.

Farquhar, John W., "How to Stop Smoking," *Medical Self-Care*, Winter, 1979/80, pages 38–49.

OTHER RISK FACTORS
Diabetes

Diabetes is a complex disease, one of the principal features of which is the body's inability to make proper use of carbohydrates (starches and sugars). It is caused by a failure of the pancreas to produce enough insulin for proper metabolism to take place, or by a defect in the action of insulin.

There are two forms of the disease: maturity-onset diabetes, the milder form, which accounts for the great majority of cases; and juvenile-onset diabetes, the more serious type and also the rarer, which appears abruptly in childhood or adolescence.

Your chances of developing either form of diabetes appear to be related to the number of diabetics in your family tree. In addition, you are more likely to get maturity-onset diabetes if you are middle-aged or older, or if you are fat. Many of those who develop the juvenile-type form of the disease have at least one diabetic parent or grandparent; however, recent research suggests that some cases of juvenile-type diabetes may be caused by a virus.

The symptoms of severe diabetes include frequent urination, extreme thirst, frequent hunger, and weight loss. The kidneys excrete large amounts of water along with the excess sugar, and this leads to the frequent urination and extreme thirst. And since diabetics cannot derive full nutritional benefit from the foods they eat, they are constantly hungry and tend to lose weight. Other symptoms are: tiring easily, itching, slow healing of infections, and blurry eyesight.

Maturity-onset diabetes usually exhibits less dramatic symptoms than the juvenile type. Its most common signs are a feeling of tiredness and weakness, body aches, numbness or tingling in the fingers or toes, blurry eyesight, and skin disorders, such as boils, carbuncles, and infections.

If you have some of these symptoms, it does not necessarily mean that you have diabetes, but it is a good idea to see your physician and make sure. He will test you for the amount of glucose in your blood or its presence in your urine.

If you have diabetes, your risk of heart attack and stroke is sharply increased, both because of diabetes' own effect on the cardiovascular system and because the disease may lead to hypertension and high blood-fat levels. The increase in risk is even greater when diabetes occurs in combination with hypertension. Diabetes is also one of the major causes of circulatory problems in the legs and feet—leading in severe cases to gangrene. (See discussion in "Circulatory Problems in the Limbs," page 79.)

You can think of diabetes as accelerating arteriosclerosis and the vascular aging process. It speeds up the "hardening of the arteries" that occurs naturally with advancing age. It affects large arteries supplying blood to such vital areas as the heart and brain, and it may also damage small blood vessels, notably those in the eyes and kidneys. Damage to blood vessels in the retina of the eye can cause hemorrhaging and blindness; in fact, diabetes is the second leading cause overall of blindness in the United States, and is the leading cause of blindness for people under age sixty-five.

Scientists don't know exactly how diabetes hastens the atherosclerotic process. One significant finding has been that, although fewer women than men suffer from cardiovascular disease, that advantage disappears for women with diabetes. Diabetic women have at least as much, perhaps more, cardiovascular disease than nondiabetic men.

Hypertension occurs much more frequently in all diabetics, both male and female, than in the nondiabetic population. Your risk of developing severe kidney disease is also increased if you have diabetes.

Diabetics also tend to have high blood-fat levels, which in turn adds to the risk of vascular complications. Diet is the first line of defense for many diabetics, particularly those whose disease is not severe, and physicians often prescribe a low-fat, low-calorie diet. There is much less concern nowadays about limiting dietary sugars or starches, and more about reducing total calories to control body weight and decreasing dietary fats to help control blood fats.

We still don't know exactly why diabetes increases the risk of cardiovascular disease; however, we do know that, because a high level of sugar in the blood does increase that risk, it's important to try to lower the blood sugar to normal. In fact, the most recent findings indicate that if this is done rigorously, at least some of the vascular complications of diabetes may be decreased. Unfortunately, it is difficult to achieve such careful control, even with insulin injections. Usually, insulin is injected once a day. The diabetic's blood sugar, on the other hand, increases sharply after each meal, and the single daily dose of insulin may not be able to counteract these peaks in blood sugar.

One new treatment approach calls for the patient to take frequent measurements of his or her blood sugar and to give him/herself frequent injections whenever necessary. Some very promising experiments have also been done with an insulin-administering pump connected to a sensing device that monitors the blood-sugar level and automatically tells the pump how much insulin to administer. Pancreas transplants are another approach, one that may prove valuable in the future for certain selected patients.

There is at present no known way to prevent diabetes. If there is a history of diabetes in your family, don't allow yourself to become overweight; if you are already overweight, reduce. It is possible, of course, to be thin and careful about your health and still develop diabetes. Regular checkups by your doctor are the best precaution.

Obesity

If you don't think being overweight increases your risk of heart attack and stroke, ask an insurance agent. Insurance companies were convinced even before medical researchers that obese people have higher mortality rates from cardiovascular disease than do slim people. They sometimes charge fat people higher premiums or require that they lose weight before they can be insured.

Obesity does most of its harm through its influence in increasing. other risk factors. If you are fat, you are more likely to have high blood pressure, diabetes, and higher levels of cholesterol and fat in your blood. If you are extremely obese, your life expectancy is significantly less than that of your slender neighbors. You are also much more likely to have hypertension. If you lose a significant amount of weight, your blood pressure is likely to drop, and you may also succeed in lowering your level of blood cholesterol and triglycerides.

You are generally considered to be obese if you are 20 percent or more over your ideal weight. (Some authorities are stricter, and set 15 percent as the cutoff point.) But, as with most risk factors, the risk tends to go up as your weight goes up, beginning somewhere slightly above ideal weight.

Through its harmful effect on other risk factors, then, obesity becomes a significant threat in itself. Weight can be difficult to control, but the benefits of lowering your weight are many. The effect on blood pressure may be particularly striking. Recent studies suggest that for every twenty-five-pound reduction in weight, an obese hypertensive on the average will experience approximately a ten-point drop in systolic blood pressure. While this might not seem like much, it is enough in many cases to reduce pressure to normal or near-normal levels in the mild hypertensive.

Though an almost obsessively diet-conscious public con-

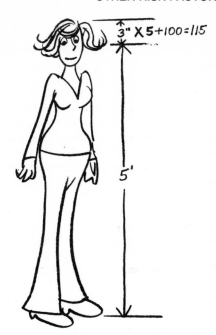

An Easy Way to Calculate Your Desirable Weight

If you are a woman, take the number of inches of your height above five feet, and multiply it by five; then add 100 pounds. For example, an approximate ideal weight for a woman five feet, five inches tall would be calculated this way: 5 (number of inches above five feet) × 5 = 25 plus 100 = 125 pounds.

If you are a man, take the number of inches of your height above five feet, and multiply it by six; then add 106. For example, for a man five feet, ten inches tall, an approximately ideal weight would be 10 × 6 = 60 plus 106 = 166.

tinues to flock from one fashionable new diet to the next, there is, unfortunately, still no miracle formula that makes it easy, safe, and fun to lose weight. If you are mildly to moderately obese, the best medical advice is still the familiar prescription: restrict your intake of calories moderately, making sure to eat a variety of nutritious foods; get regular exercise; and try to effect a permanent change in your eating and exercise habits. A gradual, steady weight loss of one to two pounds a week until you reach the appropriate weight for your height is usually safe. By selecting a variety of foods wisely, taking into account the government's recommended daily allowances for essential nutrients, you can restrict your caloric intake to as little as 1,200 calories daily and still have a healthful diet.

Regular strenuous exercise not only helps you burn up calories but also improves your physical fitness and well-being, helps you use up stored fat, and seems to have a mildly depressing effect on the appetite. Even mild forms of exercise can help you lose weight, if you don't increase the number of calories you take in at the same time. For every mile you run, or even walk, you expend approximately 100 calories. (The scientifically accurate term is "kilocalorie," which is 1,000 true calories, but we will here use the more familiar term.) For every 3,500 calories spent, there would be an expected weight loss of one pound. So, if you walked an additional two miles daily for the next year, you could expect to lose twenty pounds—assuming, of course, that you didn't eat more than you do now.

Fad diets, in which the variety of allowed foods is narrowly limited, are useless for most people in the long run and can even be dangerous. It is understandable that people who have repeatedly tried and failed to reduce their weight might become frustrated and be tempted to resort to a "quick-fix" diet. But the risks to health are often too great, and the benefits, if any, too short-lived to make fad dieting an intelligent choice. There are, however, cases where a severely restricted diet may be recommended. In the treatment of the morbidly obese—those weighing twice their ideal weight or more—a high-protein, low-carbohydrate diet (the so-called protein-sparing diet) can be an effective way to reduce weight, *but only under strict medical supervision*. Such a diet promotes rapid weight loss by facilitating the excretion of fat after it has only partly been burned up by the body's activities, and may be useful in cases where obesity is itself a life-threatening condition.

But if, like most people with weight problems, you are only moderately obese or overweight, your only chance for long-term success in controlling your weight is a permanent change in your patterns of eating and exercise.

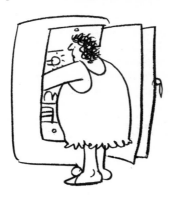

Some Strategies for Losing Weight

1. Separate eating from other activities, particularly socializing.
2. Make high-calorie foods inconspicuous or inaccessible; put them in an out-of-the-way part of your cabinets or refrigerator.
3. Stock up on low-calorie substitutes; keep them in a prominent place.
4. Prepare portions so as to make them appear larger; use smaller plates.
5. Eat slowly and chew well. Start with your salad first. Wait before taking a second portion or a

dessert; it takes time for your brain to register the fact that you have eaten.

6. Put extra food away before the meal begins.
7. Plan well-balanced meals, using familiar foods.
8. Don't skip meals. Eat three or more meals a day, each containing adequate protein.
9. Avoid crash diets. A too-rapid drop in weight can mean muscle tissue is being lost, not fat, and can lead to serious illness.
10. Budget your calories to take into account snacks and weekend eating.
11. If you find you're too hungry by mealtime, have a piece of raw vegetable, one or two soda crackers, or a small glass of vegetable juice a half-hour before mealtime.
12. Restaurants serve standard "adult" portions. Eat only what you need and leave the rest, or take it home for the next day.
13. At home, limit the places where you eat to the kitchen and/or the dining-room table.
14. Establish goals with a system of rewards (nonfood) and punishments. You will probably see fast results at first, and then a slowing down. Don't be discouraged.
15. Combine these strategies for eating less with an exercise program.

(Also see Bibliography for books on weight reduction.)

Exercise

Can exercise help you reduce your chances of suffering a heart attack? That question is a subject of continuing study— and continuing disagreement. The evidence that exercise is effective in preventing cardiovascular diseases is becoming impressive, but it's still not conclusive. Part of the problem in assessing this connection lies in the fact that heart disease has several causes. To measure accurately the effect of one contributing factor, you must control all the others very carefully. When people embark on a program of physical fitness, they frequently choose at the same time to stop smoking, change their diet, or lose weight. This makes it difficult to be sure how much of any ensuing benefits can be attributed to exercise alone, and how much to the other life-style changes.

At any rate, there are indications that exercise, by making the heart work more efficiently, may help make the consequences of a heart attack less severe. Many scientists believe exercise stimulates the growth or development of new collateral blood vessels which can compensate to some extent for blocked ones. This would mean that a physically fit person might be better able to survive a heart attack and to avoid a second one. In one study, active men were found to be three times more likely to survive a heart attack than sedentary men.

Another theory suggests that instead of stimulating collateral circulation, physical activity may enlarge existing coronary blood vessels, allowing more oxygen to pass through to the heart muscle despite any partial narrowings. This explanation may receive additional support from research on exercising monkeys currently under way at Boston University. Preliminary findings show that of two groups of monkeys fed diets high in cholesterol, the monkeys who were forced to run for a total of three hours a week on a treadmill showed much less narrowing of their arteries than the monkeys who did not exercise. The exercising monkeys also developed larger arteries, as well as a slower heart rate.

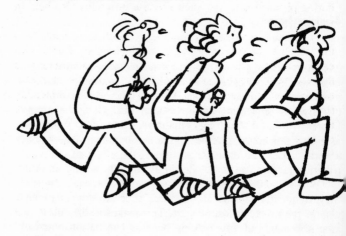

Results of another study had more good news for the nation's growing legions of runners and joggers. Researchers compared blood samples from marathon runners, joggers, and inactive people, and found that the more people ran, the higher their blood levels of high-density lipoprotein cholesterol, or HDL, a substance that is believed to reduce the risk of coronary heart disease. (See discussion of HDL, page 28.) It was the amount of running they did, rather than any difference in diet, that determined whether the subjects had high or low levels of HDLs. The study found that even joggers who averaged only eleven miles a week had significantly higher HDL levels than did inactive men, and that HDL in the blood of the runners was raised to a level that could be expected to make a significant difference in lowering their coronary risk.

Whatever the final medical verdict on the role of exercise in preventing heart attacks, one thing we *do* know is the effect exercise actually has on the work of the heart. Certain kinds of exercise programs can measurably improve your heart's efficiency, causing it to accomplish the same amount of work with less effort or expenditure of oxygen. The effect on you is to make you feel better and to increase your endurance and stamina so that you don't get winded so soon during physical activity. Such exercise programs also help in weight control.

The kind of activities that can accomplish these benefits—that is, that can improve your cardiovascular fitness—are called aerobic exercises. These are rhythmic, dynamic exercises that use major muscles repeatedly, but at a steady level, below maximum capacity. To be aerobic, an exercise must steadily supply enough oxygen to the exercising muscles for as long as the exercise is continued. Such activities include jogging, running, bicycling, swimming, rope-skipping, cross-country skiing, and brisk walking.

If you do them regularly for sufficient periods of time, these activities will produce specific physiological changes—what is known as the "training effect"—on your system. Isometric-type exercises, such as heavy weight-lifting and pushing or pulling—which serve mainly to develop muscular strength—are not effective in cardiovascular conditioning. They may even be harmful, since they can cause your blood pressure to increase appreciably—although temporarily—while they are being performed.

To achieve cardiovascular conditioning, or the training effect, you must not only do the right kind of exercises but also do the exercises for a long enough period, do them often enough, and do them at the correct level of intensity. If any one of these conditions is not met, you will achieve little or no training effect.

Exercises should be performed at least three times a week, preferably on alternate days. Every exercise session should consist of three parts: first, a warm-up of five to ten minutes, to stretch the muscles and increase their flexibility to help prevent injuries and soreness; then the aerobic exercise period itself, which should probably be limited to ten minutes in the early months of training, and gradually increased to twenty to thirty minutes after that; and finally, a cool-down period, lasting five to ten minutes, gradually decreasing the amount of effort. This helps to relax muscles that have tightened up during exercise.

The crucial part of a workout, however, is the time spent in intense activity. Here, your aim should be activity strenuous enough to cause your heart to beat at 70 to 85 percent of its maximum rate—your "target heart rate." Your maximal attainable heart rate depends not only on your age but also on your natural hereditary endowment and state of physical fitness and health. For that reason, you would ideally have it determined by a doctor—for example, in an exercise stress test. Since this is not practical for many, you might instead assume you are "average" for your age and apply the following formula for determining your target zone:

Your maximal attainable heart rate is roughly 220 minus your age. Multiply the resulting figure by .70 and by .85, to get your target zone, that is, 70 to 85 percent of your maximal heart rate, which is the zone in which you want to maintain exertion during exercise.

For example, a man of forty has a maximal heart rate of 180 (220 minus 40). If he multiplies that by .70 (126) and by .85 (153), he has determined that his target zone is between 126 and 153 beats per minute.

To determine whether your heart rate is in the target zone, you must learn to count your pulse. Press the index and middle fingers of one hand on the upturned wrist of the other hand, on the thumb side. When you find the pulse, count the number of beats that occur in exactly ten seconds, then multiply the number of beats by six, and the resulting number is your heart rate. When you start your exercise program, take it easy at first, and go slowly until you can stay comfortably within your target zone for the prescribed period. It may take weeks to reach that goal, or months. If you rush, you may hurt yourself and be unable to do any exercise at all.

Strenuous exercise is not for everyone. If you are over forty and have not exercised regularly and vigorously for a number of years, you should have a thorough checkup before starting your exercise program. Ideally—and especially if you have any of the other risk factors, such as smoking, high blood pressure, obesity, high blood cholesterol, or a family history of heart disease—that checkup should include an exercise stress test, which is an electrocardiogram taken during and immediately following exercise on a treadmill or bicycle. The older you are when starting a fitness program, the more important the exercise stress test becomes. However, because the test cannot be relied upon to be 100-percent effective in identifying existing heart problems, it should be used as one part of an overall medical appraisal of your physical condition.

Increasingly, medical centers, community hospitals, YMCAs, and other groups have been organizing exercise programs for men and women who have had heart attacks. Although such programs are still controversial, they are widespread and popular. Most experts agree that patients who have had a heart attack are better off if they carefully and gradually build up their level of activity until they are leading normally active lives, rather than retiring into semi-invalidism. Such a return to full activity should, of course, be made with caution and under the supervision of a physician.

Remember that exercise should be performed at least three times a week, and preferably more. The weekend athlete who caps a week of inactivity with a sudden burst of strenuous exercise is not doing his cardiovascular system any good, and he may be courting aches and pains, pulled muscles—or even a heart attack.

EXERCISES IN DEVELOPING CARDIOVASCULAR FITNESS

ENERGY RANGE	ACTIVITY	COMMENT
240–300 kcals/hr	Bowling	Too intermittent and not adequate to promote endurance
	Walking at 3.0 miles/hr	Adequate dynamic exercise for beginner
	Cycling at 6.0 miles/hr	As above
300–360 kcals/hr	Cycling at 8.0 miles/hr	Good dynamic aerobic exercise
	Table tennis, badminton, and volleyball	Vigorous continuous play
	Tennis—doubles	Modest benefit with continuous play
360–420 kcals/hr	Ice or roller skating	Dynamic, aerobic
420–480 kcals/hr	Tennis—singles	Can provide benefit if played 30 minutes or more continuously
480–600 kcals/hr	Jogging 5.0 miles/hr	Dynamic, endurance-building
	Downhill skiing	Usually ski runs are too short to promote endurance significantly

Oral Contraceptives and Estrogens

As you are no doubt already aware, oral contraceptives—those seemingly miraculous hormonal emancipators—are far from being an unmixed blessing. If you use the pill, you run an increased risk of, among other evils, high blood pressure, blood clots, strokes, heart attacks, and other diseases of the circulatory system. Besides being a significant risk factor by itself, the pill has also frequently turned out to be one part of an equation involving other risk factors in which the whole risk is greater than the sum of its parts.

Oral-contraceptive use represents the most important reversible cause of hypertension in women. About 5 percent of women taking oral contraceptives for prolonged periods will develop high blood pressure. When the huge number of women currently on the pill is considered—about 30 percent of fertile women—this percentage translates into a very large absolute number of women.

The longer you use oral contraceptives, the greater your chances of developing high blood pressure. However, if you do, it is usually enough simply to discontinue their use for your blood-pressure levels to return to normal—usually in about three months. If you later go back on the pill, your hypertension will return.

The risk for hypertension in women using oral contraceptives also increases with age; if you are over forty you are clearly at an increased risk. The risk is also greater if you have ever had mild hypertension or labile (highly changeable) blood pressure, if you developed toxemia or elevated blood pressure during pregnancy, if you have a family history of hypertension, if you have mild kidney disease, or if you are obese.

No one knows how oral contraceptives cause increased blood pressure, nor why only a small percentage of the women who use them become hypertensive. (Some increase in blood pressure occurs in most women who use the hormones, however.) The best current guess is that the mechanism has something to do with both constriction of the arterioles and retention of sodium by the kidneys.

Usually, the hypertension caused by oral contraceptives is relatively mild or moderate, but not always; cases of severe hypertension related to the drugs have occasionally been reported.

It is the estrogen in oral contraceptives that leads to hypertension, and estrogens prescribed for women during and after menopause can have the same hypertensive effect. The problem here is made even worse by the fact that the dosage of estrogens prescribed is frequently higher than you need to compensate for the decrease in your body's own estrogen production caused by menopause. If your blood pressure goes up while you are taking estrogen, you should be alert to the possibility that the blood-pressure increase could be due to the estrogen. If it is, your blood pressure will usually decrease to its former level within three to four months after you stop taking estrogen. In any case—whether your blood pressure has increased or not—talk to your doctor to be sure he or she is prescribing no more than the minimum dosage of estrogen you require.

If you are using oral contraceptives, or estrogens for menopause, you should have careful and repeated measurements of your blood pressure, particularly if you have a family history of high blood pressure, are overweight, or are thirty-five or older. Your blood pressure should be checked twice a year; some authorities have suggested blood-pressure checks as often as every three months during the first year of oral-contraceptive use, and every six months thereafter. Certainly you should not be on the pill if you are already hypertensive; if you develop hypertension while using oral contraceptives, you should stop taking them.

Oral contraceptives and estrogens are also linked to a marked increase in the incidence of blood clots in the veins. Blood clots occur most often in the legs (phlebitis), where they can cause pain. They can also travel to the lungs, where they cause pulmonary embolism or pulmonary infarction. (See discussion of phlebitis, page 81.)

Estimates of the degree of risk for these conditions vary. One respected study found that women taking oral contraceptives had eleven times the risk of developing venous blood clots of women not on the pill. Blood clots in the veins of premenopausal women appear to be limited almost entirely to users of oral-contraceptive drugs.

Oral contraceptives also have an important role in increasing blood fats, and they now represent the major cause of elevated levels of serum triglycerides in young women. They have been found to increase the low-density and very low-density lipoproteins and decrease the levels of high-density lipoproteins.

You also have an increased risk of stroke if you take oral contraceptives. Your risk of cerebral thrombosis, or a stroke caused by a blood clot to the brain, is ten times greater if you use the pill than if you don't. You should be aware, however, that the absolute risk is still relatively low. You may, perhaps, further minimize your risk by using pills with smaller doses of estrogen (50 micrograms or less). When you go off the pill, your risk for stroke returns to that of a nonuser.

Estrogenic drugs, including the pill, sharply increase your risk for heart attack; estimates of the increased risk range from double to fifteenfold. It is true that heart attack in women before menopause is extremely rare, and even with the increased risk caused by oral contraceptives, the absolute numbers of cases are very low. However, cigarette smoking and increased age are also risk factors, and the combination of either or both with the pill is substantially more hazardous than the combined separate effects of each. The risks rise dramatically the more you smoke, the older you are, and the longer you take the pill.

If you are a pill-user who also smokes, you are ten times more likely to die of a heart attack or circulatory disease than women who neither use the pill nor smoke. Heavy cigarette smoking, combined with the use of oral contraceptives, multiplies the risk of heart attack in premenopausal women approximately fortyfold. The estimated risk for older women (ages 38–45) who both smoke and take the pill is approximately 0.2 percent, a risk considered extemely high. When additional risk factors, such as a high blood-cholesterol level, are added to smoking and use of the pill, the risk of heart attack rises to eighty times that of a woman with none of the three risk factors.

If you are using noncontraceptive estrogen, your heart-attack risk is about nine times that of nonusers.

Where does all this leave you? If contraception is important to you, as it is to millions of others, knowing about these risks may seem to present you with an extremely difficult choice. In fact, however, it also arms you with knowledge to make the most prudent choice. If you are taking oral contraceptives, by all means have your blood pressure checked carefully at least twice a year. If you are over thirty and a smoker, consider giving up either the cigarettes or the pill. If you are over forty, if you have high blood pressure or develop it as a result of taking oral contraceptives, or if you have any of the other risk factors for hypertension, heart attack, or stroke, you should find another contraceptive method.

Behavior Type

Although scientific exploration of the role of personality traits in coronary heart disease is only beginning, physicians for centuries have suspected a correlation. The more observant among them noticed that their patients with coronary disease, particularly the younger ones, had certain traits in common that distinguished them from their unafflicted neighbors. William Harvey, the scientist who astonished the medical world in the seventeenth century by proposing that blood circulates through the body, asserted in 1628 that every disturbance of the emotions reaches the heart. Sir William Osler wrote in 1897, "I believe that the high pressure at which men live and the habit of working the machine to its maximum capacity are responsible for [arteriosclerosis] rather than excesses in eating and drinking. . . ."

Today, the proposition that psychological factors may interact with physical factors in the development of coronary heart disease is less controversial than it was twenty years ago. The

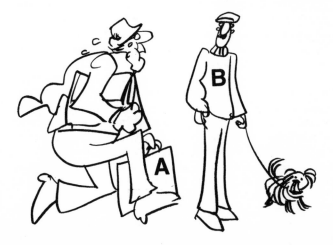

question is no longer strictly: Do personality and behavior affect coronary heart disease? but rather: How important are these factors, and how do they work?

Twenty years ago, two California cardiologists, Meyer Friedman and Ray H. Rosenman, studying psychosocial factors and their relationship to heart disease, defined a coronary-prone behavior pattern. They called those who manifest this pattern "Type A" persons, and those who don't "Type B." The coronary-prone, or Type A, person—who suffers two to three times as much heart disease as Type B—aggressively and relentlessly strives to achieve the greatest possible amount in the least possible time, impatiently steamrolling over any obstacles that may appear. The Type B person is more relaxed, unhurried, and satisfied—more unruffled by life's exigencies.

Friedman and Rosenman worked in collaboration with C. David Jenkins of Boston University, who devised a questionnaire—the Jenkins Activity Survey—that provides a practical method for measuring the presence and extent of Type A characteristics.

The evidence is becoming more and more convincing that the Type A personality is an independent risk factor in the development of coronary heart disease. Not only do Type A people have more heart attacks, but in a recent study men who were judged to be Type A by the Activity Survey were found, through coronary angiography (see explanation, page 70), to have more atherosclerosis in their coronary arteries. Surprisingly, however, the Type A personality does not appear to lead to hypertension.

Type A behavior is not simply a reaction to stress, but a persistent pattern of behavior evident in both pleasant and unpleasant life situations, provided these situations are seen by the Type A person as containing even the slightest element of challenge. Mr. Type A's personality is apparent whether he is working or on vacation, under pressure or at leisure. He seems to consider nearly all situations extremely challenging and reacts to them as if he were under great pressure to "win."

If you're a Type A, you are intensely competitive, strive for ever-greater achievement, feel pressured, and drive yourself hard. You are hasty, impatient, and restless. You place career goals above family, friends, and hobbies. You're always on the go. You have excessive motor energy that shows itself through rapid speech, clipped words and gestures, tense tight smiles, and repetitive tapping, drumming, or shaking of your hands or feet. You appear tense, you can't sit still, you can't relax, and you tend to drive, work, and eat faster than other people. Your friends might describe you as a "workaholic."

As a Type A, you are conscientious, have high values and standards, and feel people judge you by your productivity. You try to beat records and crave recognition for doing so. You like to do several things at once, and you're compulsive about getting everything done, the sooner the better.

A sense of urgency about time is almost always with you if you are Type A. Time seems to slip away too fast, and you never feel you have enough of it. You are always in a hurry, make a fetish of punctuality, and tend to become upset if you are delayed. You may, for example, lose your temper if the car ahead of you in traffic is moving too slowly.

You're not automatically Type A if your life involves a great deal of stress from a high-pressure job or family troubles. The important thing here is not whether you are under stress, but how you cope with it. The Type A person, however, thinks of himself as being under stress constantly, because he can never get where he's going fast enough or complete enough of the tasks he sets for himself.

As you can see, there are many characteristics associated with the Type A personality. It shouldn't be assumed that having *some* of them necessarily makes you a Type A person; Type B usually has a few of them too. On the other hand, you don't need to exhibit all the Type A characteristics to be a Type A. Whether you're a Type A or Type B depends on the number of characteristics of each type you possess, their intensity, and whether they coalesce into a coronary-prone behavior pattern. Interviews and written tests can help to determine whether or not you're Type A, and these tests, combined with assessments of other risk factors, can help to predict whether you have a likelihood of developing coronary heart disease.

The Type A behavior pattern, unlike the other cardiovascular risk factors, is thought to be an even greater risk factor for the *second* heart attack than the first. So if you are a Type A and you have your first heart attack, the recovery period is a good time to reevaluate your behavior and your outlook on life. You might want to try to stop judging your worth by how much you produce each day, and instead start thinking about what kind of person you are during that day—in short, to shift your concern from the quantity in your life to its quality.

Are You Type A?

- Do you constantly feel challenged to win, whether at work, at play, or in social situations?
- Do you drive yourself hard, continually striving for more productivity and greater achievement? Do you feel people judge you by what you accomplish, not by what kind of person you are?
- Are you nagged by an almost constant sense of urgency about time? Are you always in a hurry, yet still feel you can never get where you are going fast enough? Do you prefer to do several things at once?
- Is your job more important to you than your family, your friends, your other interests? Are you a "workaholic"?
- Do you set extremely high standards for yourself, and become impatient and annoyed with people whose standards appear to be lower?
- Is it difficult for you to sit still, to relax? Do you hate vacations?
- Do you drive too fast, eat too fast, talk too fast? Are your words clipped, your gestures abrupt, your smiles tense and tight? Do you drum your fingers, tap with a pencil, tap or shake your feet?
- Do you feel constantly under pressure?

The Elusive Role of Stress

Suddenly, everyone, it seems, is talking about the role of stress in various diseases, including cardiovascular disease. Yet, despite increased research activity and a great deal of discussion in the popular press, the facts remain elusive. This is partly because stress is a complex entity, difficult to define and measure with scientific precision.

Nevertheless, there are a few things we do know about stress and the cardiovascular system. There is no question, for example, that during periods of tension or anxiety, an extra burden is placed on your heart as a result of an increase in blood pressure and an increased heart rate. If you have coronary artery disease, this extra burden can cause angina. Indeed, it is well known that emotional excitement—whether of a positive or negative kind—is a common cause of angina in heart patients.

Irregular heart rhythms—arrhythmias—can also be triggered in people with heart disease by stressful situations. The risk of arrhythmias, and even of sudden death, appears to be greater under certain situations of great stress, such as the loss of a close family member. There is even some evidence to suggest that prolonged sleep deprivation or extended periods of extreme anxiety can also increase the risk for sudden death, presumably from heart disease. But though there appears to be a relationship between such disturbing events and the sudden occurrence of death in some people, it is by no means a simple cause-and-effect relationship. Its precise nature has yet to be determined.

The evidence for a link between stress and high blood pressure seems to be stronger, but even here, very little in the way of conclusive data exists. It is known that if laboratory rats are subjected to repeated stressful stimuli, such as electric shock, their blood pressure can go up and stay up. Similarly, if rats are crowded together for prolonged periods, they may develop chronic high blood pressure.

When human research volunteers are given an arithmetic problem to do in a limited period of time—a situation involving mental stress—their blood pressure rises temporarily. There is evidence that people who live in certain socially unstable urban areas—where the crime rate is high and the socioeconomic level low—tend to have somewhat higher blood-pressure levels than average. A Boston University Medical Center study of the effects of job stress on air-traffic controllers is one of the very few studies that have successfully measured the effects of stressful external events on internal bodily functions in humans. The controllers' blood pressure and heart rate were monitored in a way that enabled the men to move freely without being wired to anything outside their bodies, while trained observers recorded their work activity and emotional responses. The study found that the controllers had four times as much high blood pressure as the public at large. Over a three-year period, 14 percent of the men who had begun the study with apparently normal blood pressure experienced at least some degree of hypertension. In addition, the controllers as a group had more than their share of other stress-related diseases, such as peptic ulcers.

There is, to sum up, a widely held expectation among medical scientists that stress will turn out to be one of many interrelated factors playing a role in high blood pressure—and possibly in cardiovascular disease, too. However, the careful, scientifically valid studies that would prove this are still largely lacking. Until they are done, it is premature, most responsible experts believe, to attempt to define the role of stress.

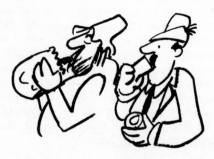

Coffee and Alcohol

If you like coffee and are afraid you are going to be advised to give it up—relax. Studies of Framingham, Massachusetts, residents have concluded that there is no reason to consider coffee a risk factor in cardiovascular disease. Coffee *had* been suspected as a risk factor because men who drink from four to seven cups a day were found to have a higher incidence of cardiovascular disease. It turned out, however, that cigarette smoking was the real culprit: the men who drank that much coffee also averaged about two and one-half times more cigarettes than non-coffee-drinkers. When heavy coffee drinkers who did not smoke were isolated in the statistics, they showed no higher prevalence of disease than those who do not drink coffee.

If you drink alcohol in markedly excessive amounts, you risk damage to your heart muscle, among many other toxic effects on your body. Heavy drinking may also cause higher than normal levels of triglycerides in the blood. And, of course, there are a lot of calories in liquor. Further, heavy drinkers seem to run a fairly high risk of developing hypertension.

On the other hand, there is no reason to believe that if you drink in moderation you run any increased risk of developing cardiovascular disease. There has even been some debate about whether drinking small amounts of alcoholic beverages might help protect against cardiovascular problems. In the Framingham study, moderate drinkers—those who consumed one to two ounces per day of hard liquor or its equivalent—were found to have a lower risk of hypertension than either abstainers *or* heavy drinkers. The blood levels of high-density lipoproteins (HDL) (see ''cholesterol'' section) may also be higher in such moderate drinkers. Thus, it is possible to conclude that a single nightly cocktail or a glass of wine might actually be therapeutic, but that anything in excess of that could be detrimental to your health.

Children and Cardiovascular Risks

Such chronic health problems as atherosclerosis and hypertension are usually seen as problems afflicting middle-aged or older people. And, for the most part, this is realistic. However, though it may take as many as twenty or thirty years for these diseases to make their presence known, they develop slowly over time, sometimes beginning quite early in life. Autopsies of American soldiers in their twenties who were killed in the Korean War disclosed evidence of significant atherosclerosis of the coronary arteries in 70 percent of the men; and in Vietnam about twenty years later, similar findings were observed. The process obviously begins early, and heart attacks can strike those in their twenties and thirties.

Clearly, the time to start doing something about preventing the development of cardiovascular diseases in your children is in their earliest years. Let's look at the risk factors again and see how they relate to the young.

Hypertension is being diagnosed in more and more adolescents and children of all ages; it has even been found in infants. Doctors don't know whether childhood hypertension necessarily leads to hypertension in the adult years, but there is increasing evidence that it might. It *is* known that hypertension tends to run in families, and that some of the children of hypertensive parents will eventually develop the disease themselves. Unfortunately, however, it is impossible to tell in advance which children these are. One clue to possible high blood pressure in children is overweight; the greater the weight, the higher the pressure is likely to be.

In a small percentage of cases, in children as in adults, blood pressure is high because of a specific physical condition, such as a malfunctioning kidney or a glandular abnormality; when the condition is corrected, the blood pressure usually falls to normal.

It is in the majority of cases, where the cause of the

hypertension is unknown, that medical science has been unsure how best to treat hypertensive children. Doctors still don't know whether it's advisable or effective to use drugs to treat children who have mild increases in blood pressure. However, children three years old and older should have their blood pressure checked annually, and those found to have sustained high blood-pressure levels should receive a systematic long-term follow-up program, with counseling on weight control, salt intake, exercise, and smoking. If elevations in blood pressure persist, drugs may also be required.

Intensive research on hypertensive children is just beginning. It may take an entire generation to get complete results, since doctors will have to watch a number of children from birth to middle age before they can come to definite conclusions. In the meantime, you and your pediatrician should be particularly watchful of your children if you or your spouse has a family history of hypertension. If you do have such a history, besides having their blood pressure checked every year, your children should have their salt intake restricted and their weight controlled. As was mentioned earlier, Americans eat a great deal more salt than they need; since salt is an acquired taste, probably the best solution to the problem is to discourage all children from developing the taste for excess salt by not adding it to their food from their earliest years. There is no cause for concern that children will fail to get the necessary amount of salt if you do this. As we have seen, prepared foods—such as bread, soup, catsup, and the like—nearly all contain added salt, and this, added to a minimal amount of salt used in cooking, will more than satisfy a child's salt needs—and an adult's, as well.

Hypercholesterolemia (high levels of cholesterol in the blood) and diabetes are both linked to family history and to diet. The extent to which they are due to heredity on the one hand and to diet on the other is difficult to establish in any single individual. However, since there is evidence of a genetic influence in the development of these two disorders, if you have a child with a family history of either one, you should be particularly alert to the possibility that these problems could develop. You should also be sure your pediatrician knows about this family history, so that he or she can be more sensitive to your child's need for monitoring, testing, and possible diet modification.

When high blood cholesterol is an inherited condition, it is known as familial hypercholesterolemia and can be a serious disease. More than 20 percent of patients who have heart attacks before age sixty have familial hypercholesterolemia, and about half of those who have the condition will experience a heart attack by the age of forty. Most people with the disease have inherited it from only one parent. However, a child unfortunate enough to inherit the trait for the disease from both parents may have extremely high levels of blood cholesterol and may suffer one or more heart attacks before he or she is twenty.

Familial hypercholesterolemia can now be diagnosed through a simple test, in which a skin sample is taken and the skin cells are studied for their ability to take up and metabolize low-density lipoproteins—an ability that is impaired in those who have the disease. In cases where both expectant parents have the disease, diagnosis can now be carried out before birth, through study of cells contained in the amniotic fluid.

The abundant evidence linking high levels of blood cholesterol with the occurrence of atherosclerotic heart disease has already been outlined in this book. We have seen how Americans, with their high rate of heart attack and stroke, have a correspondingly high level of blood cholesterol, attributable at least partially to a national diet unusually high in animal fats. We have also discussed the important effect of diabetes on cardiovascular disease, and the role of obesity in both diabetes and high cholesterol. Even knowing all this, you may find it difficult to alter the dietary habits of a lifetime, even to save your life. These dietary habits—your food likes and dislikes and your eating patterns—were formed in childhood, and childhood should be the time for establishing healthful eating patterns.

Patterns of eating established in childhood usually persist through a person's life, and if unhealthful, may influence the development and severity of atherosclerosis in later life. Too often, the dietary pattern of childhood through the teen years includes foods rich in saturated fats and cholesterol—foods like hamburgers, hot dogs, french fries, ice cream, and milk shakes. It is surprising that parents, usually so concerned about the health and sound development of their children, often take so little notice of their children's poor eating habits. Perhaps it is because those habits are not so much worse than the parents' own.

Obese parents need to be especially vigilant about their children's diet. Whether through the effects of heredity or the foods they eat—or some combination of both—the children of obese parents run a significantly greater risk of becoming obese themselves than the children of thin parents. Because people who gain extra weight in childhood find it particularly difficult to slim down as adults, an overweight child may face a lifelong struggle to control his or her weight. If you or your spouse is obese, you can help your children by remaining alert to both the quantity and quality of the foods they eat. Be especially careful to see that they don't get hooked on high-calorie foods. While watching your children's diet at home, don't forget also to check on what they are being served at the school cafeteria. If, as is sometimes the case, the lunches there are of the hot-dog-and-potato-chips school of nutrition, perhaps you could try to influence the school to revise its menu. Until it does, have your children bring their lunch from home.

Like an unhealthful diet pattern, smoking is a habit difficult to break, that is built up over the course of years. And, like bad eating habits, it frequently begins early, with a child imitating his parents. It has been found that the children of smokers are more likely to smoke than the children of non-smokers; if a child has two parents who smoke, his chances of becoming a smoker are even greater. (Besides acting as undesirable role models, parents who smoke may be directly endangering their children's health, as we have seen in the earlier discussion of the effects on children of "secondhand smoking," page 42.)

As for physical activity, there is no use exhorting your children from the depths of your armchair about the value of exercise. It is what you do, not what you say, that will have a lasting effect on their attitudes. If you are already involved in some kind of regular exercise program—jogging, swimming, sports—it would be a good idea to include your children, whenever possible.

If, instead, your children see you eating foods high in cholesterol, covering your meat with salt, eating rich desserts, allowing yourself to become fat, smoking, and spending your free time in front of the TV set instead of exercising, they are receiving a silent message from you that that is the right way to live. In order to reduce risk for your children and prevent their developing cardiovascular problems, you have to do something first about your own "risky" behavior.

No one ever said it was easy being a parent.

Circulatory Problems in the Limbs

Circulatory problems that affect blood vessels in the extremities are known collectively as peripheral vascular disease. The three most common forms are arteriosclerosis obliterans, phlebitis, and varicose veins. Less common, but of interest in our discussion, is a disorder called Buerger's disease.

As we have seen, the thickening of the walls of the blood vessels in atherosclerosis can cause heart attack when it occurs in the coronary arteries and stroke when it affects the arteries leading to the brain. The same thickening can occur in the blood vessels of the limbs—usually the legs. When it progresses to the point that blood flow in the legs is obstructed, the resulting disease is known as arteriosclerosis obliterans.

The amount of blood flowing into the leg below the obstruction is reduced, causing pain, cramps, or fatigue in the leg during exercise. This presumably is because not enough oxygen is being carried to the affected muscles. The pain disappears promptly when the leg is allowed to rest, except in the late, severe stages of the disease. (Leg cramps that occur only at night, and without exercise, are a different matter. They generally are not a serious problem and should not be confused with the symptoms of this disease.) Coldness and numbness may also be felt in the leg.

Arteriosclerosis obliterans affects people with diabetes out of all proportion to the rest of the population. The disease affects mostly older people, and men are more often affected than women. If you smoke, you are more likely to develop the disorder; cigarette smoking is second only to diabetes as a risk factor directly associated with its development. Other risk factors for the disease are the same as the other major risk factors for coronary disease. So if you are interested in prevention, you will be careful to keep your blood pressure and your blood-cholesterol level low, besides not smoking.

Patients with this problem are usually advised to stop

CONSEQUENCES OF ARTERIOSCLEROSIS
IN THE LIMBS

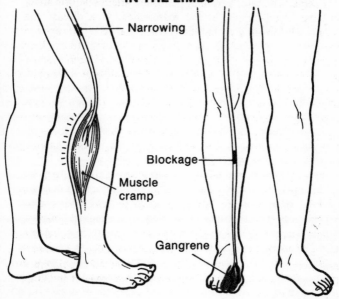

smoking, reduce any excess weight, follow an exercise program, and, if they suffer from diabetes, hypertension, or elevated levels of blood fats, to keep these conditions carefully under control. If the disease is progressive and interferes with the patient's work, surgical insertion of a bypass graft may be recommended—but generally only if the area of obstruction is limited and the arteries below it are relatively clear. In some cases, such major surgery can be avoided through the use of a new technique in which the narrowed artery is dilated by means of a special catheter, or tube, with a balloon at its tip. The catheter is fed through the artery to the area of narrowing; there the balloon is expanded with fluid, stretching the diseased artery and widening the area through which blood passes. In severe cases—when there is pain even when the patient is resting, or when ulcers or gangrene develops, and other surgical measures have been tried in vain—it may become necessary to amputate the limb.

Buerger's disease, a form of premature arteriosclerosis affecting the blood supply to the extremities, is a disease that occurs almost always in young men between the ages of twenty and forty-five. In most cases the victims are smokers, and usually they are Jewish. The disease may begin gradually, or it may come on suddenly, with gangrene developing rapidly. The symptoms are the same as in arteriosclerosis obliterans—pain or fatigue during exertion, sometimes coldness and numbness. The most critical step in treatment is getting the patient to stop smoking. If he continues to smoke, his condition will almost certainly worsen, leading possibly to amputation of the leg.

The veins, not the arteries, are the blood vessels affected by phlebitis. A vein becomes inflamed, leading to formation of a blood clot, which partially or wholly blocks the vein. Not a serious disease in itself, phlebitis can occasionally have very serious consequences: if the clot should become dislodged from the vein wall and move to the lungs (pulmonary embolism), it can interfere with essential blood circulation to the lungs. Such interference affecting large areas of the lungs can lead to death.

Using oral contraceptives increases the risk for phlebitis, as does having a malignant disease or suffering heart failure. Any long-term inactivity or immobilization, such as recovery from surgery, can increase the odds for phlebitis. That is why people taking long trips in cars or planes are advised to get out of the car or the plane seat occasionally and move around.

Treatment of phlebitis usually involves the use of anticoagulant drugs to prevent the formation of additional clots in the veins and thus minimize the risk of pulmonary embolism. In rare instances, surgery may also be required to tie off veins or otherwise prevent passage of the clot to the lungs.

Another disease affecting the veins is varicose veins, which results from the malfunction of the mechanism by which the veins carry the blood against the pull of gravity back to the heart. The veins are lined with valves which, when they are working properly, prevent any backflow of blood. If the valves are damaged and fail to close properly, the blood in the veins will tend to form pools, stretching the vein walls. The result for the sufferer may be a feeling of heaviness, aching, and fatigue in the legs, especially after a long period of standing or sitting.

Varicose veins by themselves are not serious. Usually, wearing elastic stockings and keeping the legs elevated will help prevent the pooling of blood and will be treatment enough. If these measures don't bring relief, surgery to tie off and remove the affected veins may be recommended. However, surgery is usually unnecessary.

What to Do If You Have a Heart Attack

Even if you have conscientiously tried to lower your risk factors, you can never be entirely sure of avoiding a heart attack. Some people just have heart attacks, anyway. So it's as important to know what to do when you have a heart attack as how to prevent one.

Every second counts. If you think you may be having a sudden heart attack, contact your physician and/or get to a hospital emergency room at once. Prompt and proper attention can save your life and help prevent irreparable damage to your heart.

What *are* the symptoms of a heart attack? They vary, but the usual warnings of a heart attack, as outlined by the American Heart Association, are as follows:

- Uncomfortable pressure, fullness, squeezing, or pain in the center of the chest for more than two minutes.
- Pain possibly spreading to the shoulders, neck, arms, or jaw.
- Severe pain, dizziness, fainting, sweating, nausea, or shortness of breath may also occur.
- These signals are not always present. Sometimes they subside and then return.

Get help if these symptoms present themselves. Because heart attacks often occur during physical exertion, people sometimes mistake their symptoms for muscle pulls or cramps. Others hesitate to seek help because they don't want to admit that they're ill. Still others mistakenly decide that the symptoms don't mean anything or are due to indigestion. If you are going to be wrong, be wrong on the side of caution. If you're not sure you are having an attack, call your physician or get to a hospital anyway. Don't waste valuable time trying to diagnose your pains. Avoid procrastination and don't worry about embarrassment if it turns out to be a false alarm.

The Importance of Immediate Action: CPR and Rapid-Response Emergency Care

Approximately two-thirds of the men and women who die from heart attacks do so before ever reaching a hospital or other source of medical care. Many of these deaths could be prevented through prompt, appropriate action. In recent years, increasing attention has been focused on ways to treat heart-attack victims—and others suffering sudden cardiac arrest—as soon after they are stricken as is possible. These efforts have led to development of two approaches of major public-health significance: CPR training and rapid-response emergency-care systems.

Under the auspices of the American Heart Association and the American Red Cross, hundreds of thousands of lay persons across the country have received "basic life-support training," which includes as its most important feature CPR, or cardiopulmonary resuscitation. CPR is an emergency first-aid technique for supplying breath and blood circulation temporarily to a person whose own breathing and heartbeat have stopped (and who is thus said to be suffering from respiratory failure and cardiac arrest). The sooner resuscitation is begun following cardiac arrest, the more likely the patient is to survive.

CPR is an essentially simple technique, consisting of four basic steps: first, open the victim's mouth and make sure that mouth, nose and throat are free of obstruction; then begin artificial breathing by blowing into the victim's mouth; check the pulse; if it is absent, begin a patterned pumping action on the chest over the heart to restore circulation.

While the technique is not difficult to learn, it does involve a precise coordination of mouth-to-mouth or mouth-to-nose breathing and closed-chest massage. It is not enough simply to see the technique demonstrated; you must receive training from a qualified instructor.

A course usually consists of two sessions of three or four hours each, and classes are usually held in the evening. CPR training is offered by many local Heart Association and Red Cross chapters. Your local police department, fire depart-

TECHNIQUES OF CARDIOPULMONARY RESUSCITATION

1 **Place victim flat on back on a hard surface**
Open and clear airway

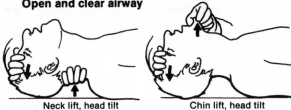

Neck lift, head tilt

Chin lift, head tilt

2 **Begin artificial breathing**

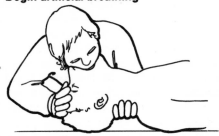

3 **Check carotid pulse**

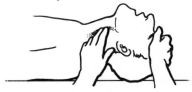

4 **If pulse is absent, begin artificial circulation**

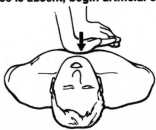

ment, or community hospital may have certified CPR instructors among their personnel.

(In addition to its value in treating sudden cardiac arrest, CPR is also useful in attempting to prevent deaths from electrocution, suffocation, drug sensitivity or overdose, and drowning.)

Though valuable, CPR by itself is not enough. Studies have demonstrated that CPR is most effective in saving lives when backed up by a community-based emergency-care system geared to reach a heart-attack victim within three to five minutes of being summoned. Such a system typically employs paramedics with advanced training for immediate response, and backs them up with mobile intensive-care units. One of the most successful such programs has been in operation in Seattle, Washington, for the past ten years. Its average response time from dispatch to arrival on the scene is only three minutes. The program, combined with the CPR training of nearly 100,000 lay residents of Seattle, has resulted in a successful resuscitation rate for heart attack victims of 40 percent. It seems likely that such systems of prehospital emergency medical care will continue to have a significant impact on heart-attack survival rates in the future.

The Warning Signs of Stroke

Before you have a major stroke, your body may warn you through one or more of the following:

- A sudden, temporary weakness or numbness of the face, arm or leg.

- Temporary difficulty in speaking or loss of speech, or trouble understanding speech.

- Sudden, temporary dimness or loss of vision, particularly in one eye.

- An episode of double vision.

- Unexplained headaches, or a change in the pattern of your headaches.

- Temporary dizziness or unsteadiness.

- A recent change in personality or mental ability.

Such symptoms may disappear again for a short period of days or weeks, then reappear either temporarily or with lasting effects as a full-blown stroke.

As in heart attack, a stroke victim should be admitted to a hospital as soon as possible. There is something you can do to assure the victim's safety until help arrives, and you should do it even before you call an ambulance. A person unconscious from stroke may have difficulty swallowing. You should clear the throat of anything that might be in it; otherwise, the victim might die from inhaling regurgitated matter.

The mortality rate for stroke victims is high, but those who survive a stroke should never lose hope. Louis Pasteur, the famous French scientist of the 1800's, carried on most of his work after suffering a major stroke. The outlook for today's stroke patient is even brighter than it used to be, particularly in hypertensive patients whose blood pressure is controlled.

Diagnostic Techniques

Because atherosclerosis develops slowly, silently, and without detectable symptoms in its early stages, its presence is not easily diagnosed. Frequently the first symptoms occur at the time of a heart attack or stroke, and by then irreversible destruction has already taken place. It's true that, before such a calamity happens, you can find out through simple tests whether you have certain risk factors, such as high blood pressure or a high cholesterol level. But only relatively complicated and costly procedures are currently available to determine whether these conditions have damaged your blood vessels.

The electrocardiogram (EKG) is a familiar test for detecting abnormalities or irregularities of the heart. It records the heart's electrical impulses on graph paper, and these tracings show whether there is an adequate supply of blood to the heart, the results of any previous heart attacks, any enlargement of the heart, and the effects of drugs. Often the EKG is administered in the doctor's office, as part of a routine physical exam. Increasingly, however, the test is proving to be more useful diagnostically when it is administered during exercise, usually on a treadmill or cycling machine. Such an exercise stress test may reveal abnormalities that would not show up in a resting EKG.

One problem with the exercise stress test is that it turns up a significant percentage of what are called "false positives"—results mistakenly indicating disease when it does not exist. Ten out of 100 men with positive test results, and 20 out of 100 women, will turn out on further investigation not to have heart disease after all. For anyone suffering chest pain, the risk of having a false positive result seems certainly worth taking. But for an apparently healthy young jogger with no chest pain, being diagnosed mistakenly as having heart disease may be damaging psychologically. For that reason, most authorities believe an exercise stress test need not be part of your routine physical examination unless you are having symptoms. They advise having the test if you have recurrent chest pain or if you wish to begin jogging or other strenuous exercise and either have other known risk factors for heart attack or stroke or are forty or over and currently leading a sedentary life.

The most important direct method for finding out the extent of atherosclerotic blockage of the arteries is through coronary angiography. This involves introducing a plastic tube into an artery in the arm or groin, leading to the heart. A dye is injected through the tube right into vessels that feed the heart muscle, and it shows up on a "cineangiogram," which is like a motion-picture X ray. The cineangiogram measures the width of the arteries in the normal and obstructed sections and shows where the blood has trouble passing. When a patient has one of the three major arteries or one of their important branches narrowed by more than 50 to 70 percent, he is defined as having significant coronary artery disease. It generally takes at least this much narrowing for blood flow to be significantly obstructed. Depending on the nature and degree of such blockage, some patients may be candidates for a coronary bypass or open-heart surgery. (See discussion in next chapter.)

The diagnosis of heart disease is currently entering a new era of noninvasive testing techniques, by which doctors are able to measure the extent of atherosclerosis and damage without the risk of invasive techniques. These noninvasive techniques include:

- radionuclear imaging, also called "thallium scan": a technique in which a small amount of a radioactive material, called thallium, containing a short-lived radioisotope, is injected into a vein, whence it travels to the heart and is taken up by the heart muscle. A scanning device measures the distribution of radioactivity and produces an image of the heart that reveals how well it is contracting and emptying the blood, and which areas of the heart may be receiving insufficient blood. When applied simultaneously with an exercise stress test, this technique not only yields more information than the stress test alone, but also produces fewer false positives. This combined approach may eventually replace the standard exercise stress test.

- ultrasound: first used to chart the ocean's floor, and known as echocardiography when it is employed to map out and measure the structure and performance of the heart. High-frequency sound waves are bounced across and through the chest, defining with remarkable clarity any structural abnormalities such as might occur in patients with congenital heart disease, valve problems, or diseases affecting the heart muscle itself.

- computerized ultrasound: among the latest and most promising advances; a noninvasive method for determining the location and extent of atherosclerotic plaques. It combines sound waves with computers to produce, from outside the body, strikingly accurate images of the walls of the arteries and any atherosclerotic lesions that may occur there. Though this procedure is currently limited to use in blood vessels near the skin's surface, such as arteries in the leg and the carotid artery in the neck, it is only a matter of time before techniques like this one will be able to provide accurate depictions of the heart without the danger and discomfort of coronary angiography.

Still further in the future, perhaps, is the fully three-dimensional imaging that would be provided by CAT (computerized axial tomography) scanning of the heart, such as is already in use for the brain and body. Because it is constantly moving, the heart presents special problems for CAT scans. However, such problems are being overcome by the use of more advanced computers, which are able to combine the information obtained from a series of rapid-sequence X rays to form an accurate three-dimensional picture of the heart. Similarly, positron tomography is being used to make detailed pictures of the heart and to study its metabolism. When perfected, these approaches are expected to revolutionize cardiology by providing physicians with a clear view from outside the body into the heart.

There is a great deal of excitement in the medical world today about the future of noninvasive diagnostic techniques. No one doubts that in the next five to ten years several new and excitingly effective methods will be developed for "seeing" into the heart and arteries. Such new techniques obviously should reduce risk and discomfort for the patient; even more significant is the capability they will give the physician to assess quickly and objectively the effectiveness of a given treatment for a given patient. With these new methods, physicians will no longer be required to wait years to see whether this therapeutic approach, or that one, leads to fewer heart attacks, strokes, or deaths.

Treatment Advances

Keeping pace with advances in diagnostic techniques has been a continuing improvement in the treatment of cardiovascular disease. As we have seen, the numbers of deaths from heart attack and stroke have dropped off remarkably in recent years. While part of this decline can no doubt be attributed to public education in prevention, another important factor has been the continuing development of more rapid and effective treatment methods.

Among the most exciting of these advances is a temporary artificial heart pump, successfully used recently at Boston University Medical Center to take over temporarily the work of a patient's heart, giving the heart time to rest and repair itself. The pump (called the left-ventricular-assist device, or LVAD) has proven to be a life-saving tool in a few cases where a patient's heart was unable to resume adequate pumping to sustain life after a heart attack or surgery. Its long-range significance, however, is as the forerunner of a total and permanently implanted artificial heart, considered by most physicians and researchers to be preferable to a human-heart transplant.

Coronary-artery-bypass graft surgery is another surgical development that has proven to be of immense value for certain types of heart patients. It is most often recommended for patients whose chronic angina is not adequately controlled by medication and interferes with their normal living. After surgery, 80 to 85 percent of such patients experience dramatic relief from pain, and in some the angina disappears completely.

In a coronary-bypass operation, doctors must construct new coronary-artery pathways to circumvent the occluded ones. For this purpose, they generally use veins taken from the patient's thigh and attach them to relatively healthy arteries around the blocked section. The operation is a serious procedure, although the risk is now relatively low at established medical centers that perform the surgery on a regular basis.

The mortality rate at such centers is usually between 1 and 5 percent.

For a time, considerable controversy surrounded the question of whether bypass surgery, besides relieving chronic angina, could also prolong life expectancy. Now, however, there is a growing body of sound evidence that, for certain classes of patients, life expectancy can be improved by performing such surgery. These include patients with disease in certain arteries—among them the left main coronary artery—who, without surgery, are at very high risk. They also include patients who have suffered cardiac arrest arising from severe arrhythmias; such patients are prone to recurrent episodes of cardiac arrest and are at sufficiently high risk of death to justify surgery. A third group is made up of patients with so-called three-vessel disease, who require triple-bypass surgery; they also appear to have a greater life expectancy if they have the surgery.

An exciting new technique (described earlier in "Circulatory Problems in the Limbs," page 79) may make major surgery unnecessary for a few patients with narrowed coronary arteries. A balloon-tipped catheter, or tube, is fed through the artery to the area of narrowing; there the balloon is expanded, dilating the narrowed segment of artery and creating a wider opening for the passage of blood. The procedure offers a potentially simple method of treatment for selected patients.

Other surgical advances include:

▪ the invention of improved artificial heart valves and artificial segments of vessels; and

▪ improvements in safety procedures for cardiac surgery that have reduced the risk of heart surgery to an impressively low level.

Of major importance in the decline of deaths from cardiovascular disease has been the massive campaigns of recent years to educate the public, especially in the area of high blood pressure. The resulting upsurge in public awareness has been accompanied by a number of important therapeutic developments. While people have begun to have their blood pressure measured regularly, scientists have been busy developing an array of drugs that lower elevated pressure so effectively that life expectancy can return toward normal.

In addition, new uses are being found for drugs already in use. Among these are the so-called beta blockers (beta-adrenergic blocking agents), such as propranolol (Inderal). The beta blockers have been used for years to decrease the rate of the heart and the amount of work it does, as well as to lower blood pressure; used in this way, they have been very useful for patients with angina. Recently researchers have shown that these drugs lower the death rate following heart attacks and reduce the rate of subsequent heart attacks.

Another group of drugs for which new uses are being discovered is the vasodilators (an example is hydralazine), traditionally used to lower blood pressure. Doctors now believe that by decreasing the heart's workload, vasodilators may also be effective in treating patients with severe heart failure.

Two new drugs hold promise for patients suffering severe heart failure. They are captopril, first tested at Boston University and recently approved for lowering blood pressure, a drug that works by decreasing the heart's workload; and amirnone, not yet approved, the first major new drug since digitalis to increase the pumping action of the heart muscle itself.

Drugs that lower blood-fat levels are another important weapon in the battle against cardiovascular disease. Several are currently prescribed—cholestyramine, colestipol, clofibrate, nicotinic acid, probucol, and others—but each has some limitation, with respect either to effectiveness or to side effects.

A promising new treatment for patients identified in the early stages of a sudden heart attack involves injecting a substance called streptokinase directly into a coronary artery obstructed by a newly formed clot. The streptokinase, a substance that occurs naturally in the body, dissolves the clot in some patients, thus opening the artery and preventing the death of heart muscle. Since its effectiveness depends on introduction of the drug soon after the clot has formed, this approach depends heavily for its success on the early recognition of a heart attack. Nevertheless, it is an exciting source of new hope for selected patients.

Meanwhile, the search continues for a drug that will prevent heart attack either by preventing disturbances in heart rhythms or by inhibiting clot formation in the coronary arteries. In a study published in early 1980, a drug then in use primarily for gout (sufinpyrazone, or Anturane) reduced dramatically the incidence of sudden death in the first few months after heart attack. However, some question still remains about the validity of these findings, and, at the moment at least, the drug is not approved for use with postinfarction patients.

Similarly, the great expectations of a few years ago that small daily doses of aspirin might head off a second heart attack have been somewhat dampened by results of a massive nationwide study that failed to support such claims. Considerably less doubt exists about aspirin's effectiveness in preventing strokes. A daily dosage of one or two aspirin tablets given to men who have had transient ischemic attacks (see page 13) appears to cut the risk of a second stroke.

Improved treatment for diabetics, who run a high risk of cardiovascular complications, is the goal of some important research currently in progress. One significant potential advance is the pump discussed in an earlier chapter (p. 49) that would administer insulin continuously, thus keeping blood-sugar levels at a consistently correct level. The pump is being developed as a possible replacement for the single daily injection now used by most patients.

As treatment methods continue to improve, another development—the introduction to the marketplace of a wide range of new food substitutes and low-fat foods—has made it easier for people to reduce such risk factors as overweight and high blood cholesterol. Many people who have been identified as being at high risk for heart attack and stroke have switched to egg substitutes and nonmeat "bacon," "hot dogs," and "hamburgers" made from vegetable products.

Such changes in dietary habits are further evidence of a new public awareness and acceptance of the individual's responsibility, in partnership with his physician, for maintaining good health and preventing untimely death from cardiovascular disease.

Boston University Medical Center:
A Leader In Heart Disease Research and Treatment

Boston University Medical Center (BUMC) has for many years been a leader in investigating the causes of heart attack and stroke, and its researchers are responsible for a number of landmark conclusions about risk factors.

Hypertension. Since the late 1940's, the research team at BUMC has pioneered the development of treatments for hypertension.

The first medication that could be counted on to lower blood pressure with any safety and consistency, rauwolfia, was introduced in the early 1950's by a Boston University team. Other drugs first used by Boston University scientists in the treatment of hypertension have included various diuretics and, recently, the medication captopril. Diuretics represented a particularly important breakthrough and continue to be the most widely used antihypertensive agents.

BUMC scientists made another extremely significant contribution to the treatment of high blood pressure by developing the "step-care" system of treatment. In this approach, now universally considered the most effective, the patient is first given a small dose of a single mild drug, most often a diuretic. If this is not enough by itself to lower the blood pressure, a second drug, aimed at a different element of the problem, is added to the treatment. And so on, in sequential steps, until the most effective combination is found.

A very broad research program currently is being carried out in hypertension at BUMC. It is directed at determining precisely which factors are involved in the causes and complications of high blood pressure and at developing new approaches for treatment that are more specifically tailored to the patient. The program has attracted international recognition, and for the past several years Boston University has been designated as a Specialized Center for Research in Hypertension by the National Heart, Lung, and Blood Institute.

The Framingham Heart Study. This long-range program was established in 1949 by the National Heart and Lung Institute to study the causes of cardiovascular diseases. When federal funding for the program was temporarily discontinued in 1970, BUMC was successful in obtaining private funds and has since had a very close working relationship with the program. Its two former directors are now professors at BUMC.

The Framingham study has been keeping track of a randomly selected group of more than 5,000 persons, aged 30 to 59 when the study began. The researchers, examining the subjects at two-year intervals, have noted which of them have developed atherosclerotic disease and have tried to determine the environmental and personal factors associated with the appearance and progression of the disease.

The study's first report, issued in 1957, helped put the word "cholesterol" into the standard American vocabulary. It concluded that people with high cholesterol levels in their blood tend to develop atherosclerotic disease. The study was also one of the first to establish the now well-accepted relationships between hypertension, smoking, diabetes, obesity, and cardiovascular diseases.

Atherosclerosis. A major research effort to clarify the causes of atherosclerosis and determine the best treatment has been under way at the medical center for the past twenty years. Investigators have induced atherosclerosis in animals through diet and have introduced new treatment methods for the problem. The team has also made major contributions to the basic understanding of how cholesterol deposits build up within the artery, and how hypertension and diabetes cause damage to the blood vessels.

Research on Coronary Heart Disease. BUMC coronary-heart-disease researchers also have earned an outstanding national reputation. They are developing and testing various ways of limiting the extent to which a heart attack damages the heart muscle. They have also shown that an artificial pump placed in the aorta of a severely ill patient may provide enough assistance to the circulation to tide the patient over the critical period following a heart attack until the severely damaged heart has had the opportunity to repair itself.

The researchers have been involved in several important large-scale national cooperative studies of heart disease. One of these was to find out whether taking aspirin regularly may reduce the risk for having a second or third heart attack (it doesn't). Another involves whether the drug propranolol has a beneficial effect in patients who have developed an acute heart attack (it does). A third is an investigation of whether coronary-artery-bypass surgery is effective in lengthening life expectancy in persons who have suffered heart attacks or who have angina. Another deals with the problem of whether reducing the levels of the major risk factors (blood pressure, blood cholesterol, and cigarette use) in adults will decrease the development of heart and vascular problems.

Investigations have also been carried out to uncover the effect of behavioral and psychosocial factors on coronary heart disease. Using a testing measure developed by BUMC scientists, studies have been conducted showing the importance of personality characteristics, Type A and Type B behavior, in the development of coronary heart disease in recovery from coronary surgery.

Drug Surveillance Program. An internationally known and unique program being carried out at BUMC monitors the long-term effects and toxicities of various medications or drugs, using data collected from a number of hospitals in the United States and various parts of the world. Among the many important new observations reported by these studies are those demonstrating the influence of oral-contraceptive drugs in increasing the risk of strokes, heart attacks, blood clots, and high blood pressure. In addition, the program has characterized the long-term side effects of blood-pressure-lowering drugs and medications for heart disease, and is constantly engaged in pursuit of evidence of new relationships among medications, life-styles, and heart disease.

The Boston University Cardiovascular Institute

Executive Committee
Aram V. Chobanian, M.D., *Director*
Robert L. Berger, M.D., *Chief of Cardiothoracic Surgery*
Jay D. Coffman, M.D., *Chief, Peripheral Vascular Disease Section*
Daniel Deykin, M.D., *Director of Medical Services, Boston Veterans Administration Hospital*
Carl Franzblau, Ph.D., *Chairman, Department of Biochemistry*
William B. Hood, Jr., M.D., *Chief of Cardiology, Boston City Hospital*
C. David Jenkins, Ph.D., *Chairman, Department of Behavioral Epidemiology*
William Kannel, M.D., *Professor of Medicine*
Norman G. Levinsky, M.D., *Chairman, Division of Medicine*
James C. Melby, M.D., *Chief, Endocrinology Section*
Thomas J. Ryan, M.D., *Chief of Clinical Cardiology, University Hospital*
Donald M. Small, M.D., *Director, Biophysics Institute*

Scientific Evaluation Committee
Aram V. Chobanian, M.D.
Edward A. Alexander, M.D., *Professor of Medicine*
Carl S. Apstein, M.D., *Associate Professor of Medicine*
Peter I. Brecher, Ph.D., *Professor of Biochemistry*
Ralph D'Agostino, Ph.D., *Professor of Mathematics*
Haralambos Gavras, M.D., *Professor of Medicine*
Christian Haudenschild, M.D., *Associate Professor of Pathology*
William Hollander, M.D., *Professor of Medicine*
Dieter Kramsh, M.D., *Associate Professor of Medicine*
Chang-seng Liang, M.D., Ph.D., *Associate Professor of Medicine and Pharmacology*
David Shepro, Ph.D., *Professor of Biology*
Graham Shipley, Ph.D., *Professor of Biochemistry*

Patient and Public Education Committee
Ann Burgess, Sc.D., *Professor of Nursing*
David Faxon, M.D., *Associate Professor of Medicine*

Michael D. Klein, M.D., *Associate Professor of Medicine*
Howard Knuttgen, Ph.D., *Chairman, Department of Health Sciences, Sargent College*
Paul Levine, M.D., *Assistant Professor of Medicine*
Joseph Stokes, M.D., *Professor of Medicine*
H. Emerson Thomas, M.D., *Assistant Professor of Medicine*
Donald Weiner, M.D., *Assistant Professor of Medicine*
Laura Wexler, M.D., *Assistant Professor of Medicine*
Irene Gavras, M.D., *Assistant Professor of Medicine*
Charles P. Tifft, M.D., *Assistant Professor of Medicine*

Bibliography

Overview

THE AMERICAN HEART ASSOCIATION. *The Heartbook*. New York: E. P. Dutton, 1980, $25.

A reference book that discusses heart and blood-vessel diseases, their diagnoses and treatment, as well as cardiovascular risk factors, warning signs, and approaches to prevention. Chapters by twenty-five nationally recognized authorities cover such areas as the physiology of exercise, diet and nutrition, hypertension, coronary heart disease, arrhythmias, and cardiac emergencies.

DEBAKEY, MICHAEL, AND ANTONIO GOTTO. *The Living Heart*. New York: McKay, 1977, $14.95.

A concise, authoritative guide to the cardiovascular system by one of America's most renowned cardiac surgeons and a leading medical expert. Discusses how the heart and blood vessels function, and what can go wrong and why. Also includes sections on cardiovascular surgery and prevention of heart disease. Richly illustrated.

Risk Factors

General

FARQUHAR, JOHN. *The American Way of Life May Be Harmful to Your Health*. New York: Norton, 1979, $9.95.

A simple, readable guide to those health habits most notably associated with heart attacks and strokes, by the director of Stanford University's Heart Disease Program. Contains material on stress, nutrition, weight control, and smoking, and includes practical, self-directed methods for lowering your risk in each of these areas.

Hypertension

GALTON, LAWRENCE. *The Silent Disease, Hypertension*. New York: New American Library, 1974, $1.95.

Discusses the nature and treatment of high blood pressure, including nondrug therapies. The section on antihypertensive drugs is a bit out-of-date. Includes useful appendices on low-sodium food and diet plans.

IRWIN, THEODORE. "Watch Your Blood Pressure." (No. 483B). Bethesda, Md.: National Institutes of Health, 1981.

One of a series of pamphlets published by the Public Affairs Committee (an independent, nonprofit, educational organization), this thirty-page booklet reviews the current state of knowledge about hypertension and the current treatments to control it.

Smoking

AMERICAN CANCER INSTITUTE "Calling It Quits" (DHEW No. NIH 79-1824), and "Clearing the Air" (DHEW No. NIH 79-1647). Bethesda, Md.: National Cancer Institute, 1979.

Booklets containing tips to help you stop smoking. Include how to cut down, avoid temptation, and avoid weight gain; also a brief list of organizations that can help you quit.

Diabetes

GOODMAN, JOSEPH I. *Diabetes Without Fear*. New York: Avon Books, 1979, $2.25.

Presents the facts about diabetes and its treatment in a lucid style. Discusses issues related to diet and to marriage and children, and includes a valuable chapter on diabetes in children. Written by a leading diabetes specialist.

Weight Control

BERLAND, THEODORE. *Rating the Diets*. New York: New American Library, 1980, $2.95.

Consumer Guide magazine has produced two valuable books—this one, and a companion volume, *Rating the Exercises* (see p. 103). Together they provide a comprehensive introduction to the respective problems of dieting and fitness, then summarize most of the current approaches. The reviews include not only books but also the major organizations active in these areas. Each book is edited by a respected expert in the field.

JEFFREY, D. BALFOUR, AND ROGER C. KATZ. *Take It Off and Keep It Off: A Behavioral Program for Weight Loss and Healthy Living*. Englewood Cliffs, N.J.: Prentice-Hall, Inc., 1977, $5.95.

Presents a behavioral program for weight loss as an alternative to dieting. Written by two clinical psychologists, who use a series of behavioral self-control techniques to help you identify and change your eating habits. Includes techniques for building and maintaining motivation and social support, methods for managing your feelings and your food-buying habits, and instructions on how to keep food and activity diaries. Also contains valuable advice for improving a child's eating patterns.

(Other, similar books in the same vein are: Mahoney, Michael and Kathryn. *Permanent Weight Control: A Total Solution to the Dieter's Dilemma*. New York: W. W. Norton, 1976, $11.95.; and Stuart, Richard. *Act Thin, Stay Thin*. New York: W. W. Norton, 1976, $11.95.

WOLF, JURGEN, AND DEWEY LIPE. *Help for the Overweight Child*. New York: Penguin Books, 1980, $2.95.)

A short paperback that describes how children develop weight problems, then tells parents how they can help their overweight child—first by identifying his or her specific eating habits and then by providing a number of positive incentives for weight loss, along with guidance about appropriate diet. Includes useful information on exercises, healthful snacks, and the caloric content of common foods.

Exercise

COOPER, KENNETH H. *The New Aerobics*. New York: Bantam Books, 1970, $2.75.

An update of Dr. Cooper's original aerobics program, providing details for a graduated exercise program. Exercise levels are divided by age and type of exercise—walking, running, swimming, handball, etc. Includes sections on aerobics for women and on exercising indoors.

DONALDSON, RORY, ed. *Guidelines for Successful Jogging*. Washington, D.C.: The National Jogging Association, 1977, $3.95.

A short book that guides the inexperienced but motivated person through the steps necessary to develop a successful running program. Contains a particularly good section on muscle-stretching exercises; also has information on equipment and on running in various kinds of weather.

KUNTZLEMANN, CHARLES T. *Rating the Exercises*. New York: New American Library, 1980, $2.50.

Described above under "Berland, Theodore. *Rating the Diets*."

SHEPRO, DAVID, AND HOWARD KNUTTGEN. *Complete Conditioning*. Reading, Mass.: Addison Wesley, 1975, $4.95.

Subtitled "The No-Nonsense Guide to Fitness and Good Health." The authors, professors of biology and physiology, respectively, at Boston University, believe the cornerstone of cardiovascular health is proper diet and exercise. Divided into sections on the physiology of exercise, how to start an exercise program, good nutrition, and weight control. Includes an extended and informative glossary of terms related to health and fitness.

ZOHMAN, LENORE R. "Beyond Diet—Exercise Your Way to Fitness and Health." Englewood Cliffs, N.J.: Best Foods, 1974.

An excellent booklet that describes why you should maintain cardiovascular fitness, and how to determine whether an exercise program will be beneficial. Outlines activities that improve heart health, and includes sections on the use of a stationary bicycle and on rope-skipping.

Behavior and Stress

THE BLUE CROSS ASSOCIATION. "Stress." Chicago: The Blue Cross Association, 1974.

A booklet containing a series of brief articles by authorities in the field of stress. Explains what stress is, and how it operates in different age groups and social settings. Also includes a section on relaxation exercises.

FRIEDMAN, MEYER, AND RAY ROSENMAN. *Type A Behavior and Your Heart*. New York: Fawcett, 1978, $2.50.

Presents the authors' case for the importance of Type A behavior patterns in the development of cardiovascular disease. Includes chapters describing the Type A personality and drills for altering this behavior pattern.

Nutrition

DEUTSCH, RONALD. *Realities of Nutrition*. Palo Alto: Bull Publishing Co., 1976, $8.50.

A clear and lucid presentation of a complex subject by a noted science writer. Discusses basic principles of energy, exercise, and the body's storage of fat; explains the various nutrients—carbohydrates, fats, proteins, and vitamins—the principles of weight control, and the composition of a balanced diet. Includes discussions of such controversial topics as natural foods and food additives.

MAYER, JEAN. *A Diet for Living*. New York: Pocket Books, 1976, $1.95.

Written by an internationally respected nutritionist. Uses a question-and-answer format to provide concise information on the nutritional issues Mayer considers most important and/or most confusing to the public. Includes extensive information on the facts and fiction about nutrition, weight and well-being, the marketplace and the kitchen.

Cookbooks

CLAIBORNE, CRAIG, AND PIERRE FRANEY. *Craig Claiborne's Gourmet Diet*. New York: Times Books, 1980, $9.95.

Contains more than two hundred low-calorie, low-salt recipes developed for himself by the world-renowned food writer and gourmet after he learned he suffered from hypertension. The authors have been particularly inventive in finding substitutes that enhance the flavors of food. Each recipe lists the number of calories and the sodium, cholesterol, and fat content.

EISHELMAN, RUTHE, AND MARY WINSTON, editors. *The American Heart Association Cookbook*. Hardcover edition—New York: McKay, 1979, $12.95. Paperback—New York: Ballantine, 1979, $2.95.

A compilation of recipes—from appetizers and soups to main dishes and desserts—from Heart Association chapters across the country. The emphasis is on nutritious, fat-controlled, low-sugar meals. Each recipe also includes approximate caloric intake per serving. Included are vegetarian meals, fat-cholesterol charts, and an introduction that discusses what makes a diet healthful for your heart.

MARGIE, JOYCE DALY, AND JAMES C. HUNT. *Living with High Blood Pressure—The Hypertension Diet Cookbook*. Radnor, Pa.: Chilton, 1979, $13.95.

Useful not only for hypertensives who must maintain a low-sodium diet but also for anyone interested in reducing salt and saturated fat in his or her diet. Contains an introductory description of hypertension and its treatment by Dr. Hunt (who is dean of the University of Tennessee School of Medicine), as well as sections on food plans, menus, nutritive-value charts, and the addresses of places where you can buy special low-sodium products.

Glossary

A number of the following definitions have been drawn wholly or in part from *A Handbook of Heart Terms*, published by the U.S. Department of Health, Education and Welfare, Public Health Service, National Institutes of Health.

ADRENAL GLAND—Complex gland located just above each kidney, which secretes a variety of hormones concerned with salt balance and several metabolic and sexual functions. It also secretes noradrenalin (norepinephrine) and adrenalin (epinephrine), which influence constriction of small blood vessels, heart rate, blood pressure, and reaction to stress.

AEROBIC EXERCISE—Any rhythmic, repetitive, dynamic activity, such as running, bicycling, and swimming, is generally aerobic.

ANGINA PECTORIS or ANGINA—Literally, chest pain. A condition in which the heart muscle receives an insufficient blood supply, causing pain in the chest and often in the left arm and shoulder. Commonly results when the arteries supplying the heart muscle (coronary arteries) are narrowed by atherosclerosis.

ANGIOGRAPHY—X-ray examination of blood vessels following injection of an opaque fluid into the bloodstream.

AORTA—The main trunk artery that receives blood from the left chamber of the heart. Leading off from it are many lesser arteries, which conduct blood to all parts of the body.

AORTIC ANEURYSM—A ballooning-out of the wall of the aorta, due to weakening of the wall by disease, traumatic injury, or an abnormality present at birth.

ARRHYTHMIA—Any variation from the normal rhythm of the heartbeat.

ARTERIOLES—The smallest arterial vessels, constituting the terminal branching "twigs" of the arteries. They conduct blood from the arteries to the capillaries.

ARTERIOSCLEROSIS—Commonly called hardening of the arteries. This is a generic term that includes a variety of diseases characterized by thickening and loss of elasticity of artery walls.

ARTERIOSCLEROSIS OBLITERANS—Disease in which atherosclerotic thickening in the blood vessels of the limbs—usually the legs—obstructs blood flow, causing pain, cramps, or fatigue in the limb during exercise.

ARTERY—A blood vessel which carries oxygenated blood away from the heart to the various parts of the body. (An exception, though, is the pulmonary artery, which carries unoxygenated blood from the heart to the lungs for oxygenation.)

ATHEROSCLEROSIS—A type of arteriosclerosis in which the inner layer of the artery wall is thickened by cellular material and deposits of several substances, particularly fats. These deposits (called atheromata) may decrease the diameter of the internal channel of the vessel.

ATHEROSCLEROTIC BRAIN INFARCTION—Blockage of the blood vessels to the brain, causing death to the section of the brain deprived of oxygen.

BETA BLOCKERS (beta-adrenergic blocking agents)—Drugs which, by blocking the normal response of the heart and blood vessels to nerve impulses transmitted by the adrenergic nervous system (more or less the same as the sympathetic nervous system), tend to decrease the heart rate and the vigor of heart contractions, as well as to lower blood pressure. Often used to treat angina pectoris. Propranolo 1 (Inderal), metoprolol (Lopressor), nadolol (Corgard), timolol (Blocadren), and atenolol (Tenormin) are the five beta blockers currently approved for use by the FDA.

BLOOD PRESSURE—The force the flowing blood exerts against artery walls. The two pressures that are measured are the upper, or systolic, pressure, which occurs each time the heart contracts and pumps blood into the aorta; and the lower, or diastolic, pressure, which occurs each time the heart relaxes between beats and refills with blood flowing in from the large veins.

CAPILLARIES—Extremely narrow tubes forming a network between the arterioles and the veins. The walls are composed of a single layer of cells through which oxygen and nutritive materials pass out to the tissues, and carbon dioxide and waste products are admitted from the tissues into the bloodstream.

CARDIAC ARREST—Cessation of the heartbeat. No longer always fatal, thanks to techniques for stimulating the heart to start it beating again under certain circumstances (See Cardiopulmonary Resuscitation.)

CARDIOPULMONARY RESUSCITATION (CPR)—An emergency first-aid technique for supplying breath and blood circulation temporarily to a person whose own breathing and blood circulation have stopped.

CARDIOVASCULAR DISEASE—Any disease of the heart or blood vessels.

CEREBRAL INFARCTION—Death of brain tissue due to interruption of its blood supply.

CEREBRAL THROMBOSIS—A stroke caused by a blood clot to the brain.

CHOLESTEROL—A fatlike substance found in animal tissue, including the blood. In blood tests the normal level for Americans is assumed to be between 180 and 220 milligrams per 100 cubic centimeters. A higher level is often associated with high risk of coronary atherosclerosis.

COLLATERAL CIRCULATION—Circulation of blood provided from nearby smaller vessels when a main vessel has been blocked up.

CORONARY ANGIOGRAPHY—A diagnostic method in which a dye is injected into vessels that feed the heart muscle. The dye shows up on a motion-picture X ray, outlining the arteries and showing where any abnormalities in blood flow may occur.

CORONARY ARTERIES—Arteries arising from the base of the aorta, which conduct blood to the heart muscle. They, and the network of vessels branching off from them, come down over the top of the heart like a crown (corona).

CORONARY-BYPASS SURGERY—Surgery to improve the blood supply to the heart muscle caused by narrowing of the coronary arteries. Involves constructing new coronary-artery pathways to circumvent, or bypass, the narrowed ones—

generally using veins or arteries taken from other parts of the body, such as the thigh, and grafting them onto relatively healthy arteries around the blocked section.

CORONARY HEART DISEASE—Disease of the heart occurring as a result of impairment in its blood supply. The usual cause is atherosclerosis of the coronary arteries with resultant reduction of blood supply to the heart muscle. Heart attacks or angina may result.

DIABETES—A disorder in which the body is unable to metabolize sugars properly, usually because the pancreas is failing to produce enough insulin for the proper metabolism to take place.

DIASTOLIC BLOOD PRESSURE—The blood pressure during the period of the relaxation of the heart; the lowest pressure observed during the heart cycle.

DIURETIC—A medicine that promotes the excretion of salt and water in the urine.

ELECTROCARDIOGRAM—Often referred to as EKG or ECG. A graphic record of the electric currents produced by the heart.

EMPHYSEMA—A disease of the lung marked by distension and frequently associated with impairment of lung function.

EPIDEMIOLOGY—The study of the circumstances surrounding the development of disease in a given population.

ESSENTIAL HYPERTENSION—Elevated blood pressure of unknown cause. Sometimes called primary hypertension.

EXERCISE STRESS TEST—An electrocardiogram taken while the patient is exercising—usually jogging on a treadmill, walking up and down a short set of stairs, or pedaling a stationary bicycle.

FALSE POSITIVE—Medical-test results mistakenly indicating disease when it does not exist.

FIBRILLATION—A kind of cardiac arrhythmia in which the contractions of the heart muscle are irregular and uncoordinated because individual muscle fibers are contracting independently.

HARDENING OF THE ARTERIES—See Arteriosclerosis.

HEART ATTACK—Damage or death of heart muscle due to insufficient blood supply to the heart.

HEART FAILURE—A condition in which the heart is unable to pump enough blood to maintain normal circulation. Often leads to congestion in the body tissues; fluid accumulates in the abdomen and legs and/or in the lungs (pulmonary edema).

HIGH-DENSITY LIPOPROTEIN (HDL)—One of two of the major types of lipoproteins normally found in the blood that have opposite effects on the arteries—the other being low-density lipoprotein (LDL). HDL appears to protect against atherosclerosis; persons whose HDL cholesterol is relatively high have less risk of developing coronary heart disease.

HYPERCHOLESTEROLEMIA—An excess of a fatty substance called cholesterol in the blood.

HYPERTENSION—Commonly called high blood pressure. Elevation of blood pressure above the normal range.

INCIDENCE—The number of new cases of a disease developing in a given population during a specified period of time, often a year.

INFARCTION—Damage to, or the death of, an area of tissue as a result of receiving an insufficient blood supply. Myocardial infarction is injury to an area of heart muscle due to the interrupted flow of blood through the coronary artery which normally supplies it.

INSULIN—An essential hormone produced by the islands (or bodies) of Langerhans in the pancreas, which facilitates the utilization of sugar in the body.

INTRACRANIAL HEMORRHAGE—Bleeding into the substance of the brain that occurs when disease-weakened or congenitally weak blood vessels rupture.

ISCHEMIA—A local, usually temporary deficiency of blood supply in some part of the body, often caused by narrowing or obstruction of a blood vessel supplying that part.

LABILE BLOOD PRESSURE—Highly changeable blood pressure.

LIPOPROTEIN—A complex substance consisting of lipid (fat) and protein molecules bound together. Lipids do not dissolve in the blood, but must circulate in the form of lipoproteins.

LOW-DENSITY LIPOPROTEIN—A major lipoprotein normally found in the blood which appears to promote the development of atherosclerosis; persons whose LDL cholesterol levels are high have a greater risk of developing coronary artery disease.

MYOCARDIAL INFARCTION—The damage or death of an area of the heart muscle (myocardium) resulting from a reduction in blood supply to that area.

OBESITY—An excess of body weight beyond physical and skeletal requirements due to an accumulation of excess fat. You are generally considered to be obese if you are 15 to 20 percent or more above your ideal weight.

OCCLUSION—Blockage or obstruction.

PANCREAS—The large elongated gland found in the abdomen behind the stomach, which secretes digestive enzymes and the hormone insulin.

PERIPHERAL VASCULAR DISEASE—Collective name for circulatory problems that affect blood vessels in the arms and legs. The three most common are arteriosclerosis obliterans, phlebitis, and varicose veins.

PHLEBITIS—Disease in which a vein—usually in the leg—becomes inflamed, often leading to formation of a blood clot, which partially or wholly blocks the vein.

PLAQUE—A deposit of fatty (and other) substances in the inner lining of the artery wall, characteristic of atherosclerosis. Also called atheroma.

POLYUNSATURATED FAT—A fat so constituted chemically that it is capable of absorbing additional hydrogen. These fats are usually liquid oils of vegetable origin, such as corn oil or sunflower oil.

RADIOISOTOPES—Radioactive forms of elements.

RISK FACTORS—Those physical conditions or life habits that are thought to influence one's likelihood of suffering cardiovascular diseases.

SATURATED FAT—A fat so constituted chemically that it is not capable of absorbing any more hydrogen (hydrogenated). These are usually the solid fats of animal origin, such as the fats in milk, butter, meat, etc.

SERUM—The fluid portion of blood that remains after the blood has clotted. It is different from plasma, which is the cell-free liquid portion of unclotted blood.

SODIUM—A mineral essential to life, found in nearly all plant and animal tissue. Makes up nearly half of table salt (sodium chloride). Appears to be important in the development of high blood pressure.

SPHYGMOMANOMETER—An instrument for measuring blood pressure.

STRESS—Bodily or mental tension caused by physical, chemical, or emotional factors. Though often thought of in terms of mental anxiety, stress can refer to physical exertion as well.

STROKE—An impeded blood supply to some part of the brain, and resultant change in brain function, generally caused by:
    (1) a blood clot forming in the vessel (cerebral thrombosis);
    (2) a rupture of the blood-vessel wall (cerebral hemorrhage);
    (3) a blood clot or other material originating from another part of the vascular system that flows to the brain and obstructs a cerebral vessel (cerebral embolism); or
    (4) pressure on a blood vessel, as by a tumor.

SYSTOLIC BLOOD PRESSURE—The peak blood pressure during the period of the contraction of the heart.

TRAINING EFFECT—Certain specific physiological changes, including measurable improvement of the heart's efficiency, resulting from the regular performance of aerobic exercises (for example, running, swimming, and bicycling) for a certain period of time, with a certain frequency and at a certain level of intensity.

TRANSIENT CEREBRAL ISCHEMIA—A "little stroke," caused by partial blockage of blood vessels or insufficient blood flow to the brain, which may precede a full-blown stroke. Can cause slurred speech, dizziness, numbness, or weakness of the limbs that may pass in a few minutes or a few hours.

TRIGLYCERIDES—An important group of body fats differing from cholesterol, which may also increase the predisposition to atherosclerosis when elevated levels are present in the blood.

TYPE A BEHAVIOR—A behavior pattern thought by some cardiologists to be a risk factor for heart attack. Characterized by competitiveness, aggressiveness, and a sense of urgency about time. Type B persons are more easygoing and unhurried, and more easily satisfied.

ULTRASOUND—High-frequency sound vibrations, not audible to the human ear, which can be used to map out and measure the structure and performance of the heart.

VARICOSE VEINS—Swollen veins, found most often on the legs, resulting from the malfunction of the mechanism by which the veins carry the blood against the pull of gravity back to the heart.

VASODILATORS—Drugs such as nitroglycerin and hydralazine (apresoline) that cause a relaxation of the muscles of the arterioles. Long used to lower blood pressure, they are now believed effective in treating severe heart failure.

VEIN—A blood vessel which carries unoxygenated blood from various parts of the body back to the heart. (The pulmonary vein, though, conducts freshly oxygenated blood from the lungs back to the heart.)

INDEX

ABOUT THE AUTHORS

ARAM V. CHOBANIAN, one of the most highly respected authorities on hypertension in the country, is director of the Cardiovascular Institute of Boston University Medical Center. He is a professor of medicine at Boston University School of Medicine, where he also directs the Hypertension Specialized Center of Research.

Chobanian has been chairman of both the National Heart, Lung and Blood Institute's Advisory Committee on Hypertension and Arteriosclerosis and of the Food and Drug Administration's Cardiovascular and Renal Advisory Committee.

A graduate of Harvard Medical School, he is a member of several prestigious societies, including the Association of American Physicians and of the American Society of Clinical Investigation. His name consistently appears on published lists of the best physicians in America. He is the author of approximately 150 articles on cardiovascular diseases.

LORRAINE W. LOVIGLIO, former editor for academic affairs at Boston University Medical Center, is an award-winning journalist who has written extensively on medical subjects for the general reader.